ALLE ZEIT WACH
SJ
1842

BG Chemie

# Toxicological Evaluations

## 3 Potential Health Hazards of Existing Chemicals

Springer-Verlag
Berlin Heidelberg New York
London Paris Tokyo
Hong Kong Barcelona
Budapest

Berufsgenossenschaft
der chemischen Industrie
Gaisbergstraße 11
W-6900 Heidelberg 1, FRG

ISBN 3-540-54331-7 Springer Verlag Berlin Heidelberg New York
ISBN 0-387-54331-7 Springer Verlag New York Berlin Heidelberg

Library of Congress Cataloging-in-Publication Data. (Revised for volume 3). Toxicological evaluations. Includes biblographical references and index. 1. Toxicity testing. I. Berufsgenossenschaft der Chemischen Industrie. [DNLM: 1. Hazardous Substances – toxicity. WA 465 T7549] RA1199.T678 1990 615.9'07 90-10020
ISBN 3-540-54331-7 (alk. paper)
ISBN 0-387-54331-7 (alk. paper)


Printed in Germany



Typesetting, printing and bookbinding: Brühlsche Universitätsdruckerei, Giessen
51/3130-543210 – Printed on acid-free paper

# Preface

As part of its programme for the prevention of health hazards caused by industrial work substances, the Berufsgenossenschaft der chemischen Industrie (BG Chemie) began in 1977 to investigate the toxicity of those substances which are widely used, have many different applications and are suspected of being dangerous to health, in particular those having long-term effects on health. The investigations consist of a literature search and – depending on the results – commissions of experimental studies. It is hoped by means of this testing to close gaps in our knowledge and to increase the scientific validity of the required risk assessments. The results of the toxicological investigations carried out by BG Chemie, and the resulting substance assessments have been published in German since 1987 in the form of „Toxikologische Bewertungen" („Toxicological Evaluations").

In order to make this useful information internationally available, the third volume (containing individual evaluations of 13 substances) of the series is now being published in English, the first volume of which was published in October 1990. Because of the short time between publishing volume 1, 2 and 3, printing of the „Introduction" (consisting of a general overview of the programme, lists with names of people involved as well as substances under investigation) was abandoned in volumes 2 and 3. If more detailed information is required, see volume 1 or contact BG Chemie at first hand.

The publication of further individual evaluations and, if necessary, reassessments of previously published evaluations is planned.

BG Chemie hopes that, for many people working in the chemical industry, this information will be of practical help in assessing hazards to health at the workplace.

# Contents


| Name of substances | CAS-No. | Page |
|---|---|---|
| Bromoform | 75-25-2 | 1 |
| Diethyl carbamoyl chloride | 88-10-8 | 19 |
| o-Chlorobenzotrifluoride | 88-16-4 | 27 |
| Chloro acetic acid methyl ester | 96-34-4 | 33 |
| m-Chlorobenzotrifluoride | 98-15-7 | 41 |
| Terephthalic acid | 100-21-0 | 47 |
| Isopropyl ethylene glycol ether | 109-59-1 | 61 |
| Phenylglycidyl ether | 122-60-1 | 73 |
| Thiram | 137-26-8 | 91 |
| Methoxyacetic acid | 625-45-6 | 131 |
| o-Chlorobenzotrichloride | 2136-89-2 | 147 |
| Diglycidyl ether | 2238-07-5 | 155 |
| p-Chlorobenzotrichloride | 5216-25-1 | 167 |
| Compound chemical index vol. 1–3 | | 179 |

# Bromoform

## 1. Summary and assessment

In contrast to chloroform, studies on the distribution, elimination and metabolism of bromoform are not available. In metabolic studies relating to a separate question it is found that bromoform, like iodoform and, in small amounts, chloroform, can be metabolised in vitro and in vivo to carbon monoxide.

On single administration, bromoform shows itself to be mildly toxic ($LD_{50}$ oral 1147–1550 mg/kg, $LD_{50}$ dermal >2000 mg/kg) and produces ataxia, somnolence, narcosis and haemorrhages of the internal organs of experimental animals. Subacute (oral, dermal, inhalation) and subchronic (oral) toxicity data in rodents indicate that bromoform can produce reversible changes in the liver and kidneys and the liver and thyroid gland, respectively.

Bromoform has a very slight, reversible, irritant action on the skin and eyes of rabbits.

In the Salmonella/microsome test, bromoform has given negative, equivocal and positive results in the presence or absence of a metabolic activation system. Bromoform is mutagenic in mouse lymphoma cells *in vitro* and in the Drosophila test *in vivo*, and it induces micronuclei *in vitro* and sister chromatid exchange *in vivo*. In contrast, no chromosome aberrations are induced either *in vitro* or *in vivo*.

Limited 24-week studies in mice involving intraperitoneal injection provide some indication of possible carcinogenic activity for bromoform. Preliminary results of a long-term (24-months) oral study in rats have given no evidence of carcinogenicity (evaluation of the histopathological findings is still outstanding). In further long-term (103-wk) oral investigations in rats and mice, there is "some evidence" of carcinogenic activity in male rats and "clear evidence" of carcinogenic activity in female rats, whilst in the mice there are no consistent indications. On the basis of these findings, the possibility that bromoform is carcinogenic cannot be excluded.

Bromoform shows itself to be slightly embryotoxic in rats (sternebrae aberrations, interparietal deviations).

In the mouse, bromoform suppresses the humoral and cellular immune response.

In man, accidental exposure to bromoform produces breathing difficulties, cyanosis, increased pulse rate and loss of consciousness.

In the USA the threshold limit value is given as 5 mg/m$^3$ TLV 1988–1989).

## 2. Name of substance

| | | |
|---|---|---|
| 2.1 | Usual name | Bromoform |
| 2.2 | IUPAC-name | Tribromomethane |
| 2.3 | CAS-No. | 75-25-2 |

## 3. Synonyms, common and trade names

Methenyltribromide

## 4. Structural and molecular formulae

4.1 Structural formula

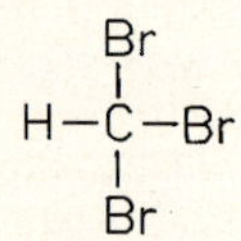

4.2 Molecular formula $CHBr_3$

## 5. Physical and chemical properties

| | | |
|---|---|---|
| 5.1 | Molecular mass, g/mol | 252.75 |
| 5.2 | Melting point, °C | 8.3 (ACGIH, 1988) |
| 5.3 | Boiling point, °C | 149.5 (ACGIH, 1988) |
| 5.4 | Vapour pressure, hPa | 6.668 (at 20 °C) (ACGIH, 1988) |
| 5.5 | Density, g/cm$^3$ | 2.889 (at 20 °C) (ACGIH, 1988) |
| 5.6 | Solubility in water | 0.1 g/100 g water (at 20 °C) (ACGIH, 1988) |
| 5.7 | Solubility in organic solvents | soluble in alcohol, ether, benzene, chloroform |
| 5.8 | Solubility in fat | no information available |
| 5.9 | pH-value | no information available |

5.10 Conversion factor

1 ppm $\hat{=}$ 10.35 mg/m³
1 mg/m³ $\hat{=}$ 0.097 ppm
(at 25 °C and 1013 hPa)
(ACGIH 1988),

## 6. Uses

Separation of inorganic mixtures; synthesis in organic chemistry (Neumüller, 1979).

## 7. Experimental results

### 7.1 Toxicokinetics and metabolism

In a study by Binz (1891) it was reported that after inhalation exposure or subcutaneous injection of bromoform in rabbits, bromide appears in the urine.

Unlike for chloroform, studies on the distribution, elimination and metabolism of bromoform are not available, but it can be assumed that this chemical is metabolised in a similar way. In metabolic studies investigating a specific question it was found that bromoform, like iodoform and to a lesser extent chloroform, can be metabolized to carbon monoxide *in vivo* and *in vitro* (Ahmed et al., 1977; Anders et al., 1978). It was concluded from these results that bromoform is probably metabolised by cytochrome P450-dependent mixed-function oxidases in the liver to carbon monoxide. *In vivo*, carbon monoxide production (and thereby carboxyhaemoglobin formation) was dose-dependent. The administration of $^{13}$C-labelled bromoform leads to increased formation of radiolabelled carbon monoxide with increasing dose level (Stevens and Anders, 1979).

### 7.2 Acute and subacute toxicity

The oral $LD_{50}$ value of bromoform was determined in male (30–35 g) and female (25–30 g) ICR-Swiss mice. The test substance was dissolved im Emulphor : alcohol : saline (1 : 1 : 8) and administered by stomach tube to the fasted animals (0.01 ml/g body weight; no further details). Doses of between 500 and 4000 mg/kg were administered to ten females and ten males per dose. The observation period was 14 days. For male mice an $LD_{50}$ value of 1400 mg/kg was reported (95% confidence limits, 1205–1598 mg/kg) and for female mice a value of 1550 mg/kg (95% confidence limits, 1165–2062 mg/kg). The animals died between the first and ninth day after administration. Symptoms of bromoform toxicity observed at doses of over 1000 mg/kg were ataxia, sedation (duration about 4 hours) and narcosis. All animals which died during the experiment were dissected and macroscopically examined. The livers exhibited fatty infiltration, the kidneys were pale, and the adrenal glands, lungs and brain showed haemorrhages (Bowman et al., 1978).

Kutob and Plaa (1962) investigated the subcutaneous $LD_{50}$ of bromoform in male Swiss-albino mice (starting weight 20–30 g). The test substance was made up in olive oil. The individual doses (no further details) were administered in a volume of 0.05 ml/10 g body weight. The observation period was 10 days. The $LD_{50}$ was determined as 7.2 mmol/kg (corresponding to about 1822 mg/kg). The 95% confidence limits lay between 6.4 and 8.1 mmol/kg, corresponding to approximately 1618–2047 mg/kg.

Chu et al. (1980, 1982 a) studied the acute oral toxicity of bromoform in male and female Sprague-Dawley rats (starting weight 150–200 g). Five doses of 546–2100 mg/kg were used. Each dosage group comprised ten males and ten females. The observation period was 14 days. The $LD_{50}$ values were determined as 1388 mg/kg for male rats (95% confidence limits, 1167–1693 mg/kg) and 1147 mg/kg for female rats (95% confidence limits, 890–1524 mg/kg). Symptoms of bromoform toxicity were described as follows: piloerection, sedation, loss of muscle tone, ataxia, prostration and hypothermia. The liver and kidneys of the animals were congested and enlarged. A reduction in the protein content of the liver occurred in male rats, but not in females. In female rats, an increase in microsomal aniline hydroxylase was observed. On haematological examination, a decrease in the number of lymphocytes was seen mainly in the females.

Two rabbits survived a single application of 2000 mg/kg undiluted bromoform to the intact skin under a cuff for 24 hours, but they showed lethargy and slight weight loss (Torkelson and Rowe, 1981).

Dykan (1965) subjected rabbits (sex and strain not given) to a single inhalation exposure of 11–13 mg/l (exposure time not given). Disturbances of the central nervous system were observed. No further details of this experiment are available.

Munson et al. (1982) investigated the subacute toxicity of bromoform on oral administration to male and female CD1 mice. The chemical was dissolved in water with 10% Emulphor. Volumes of 0.01 mg/g body weight were used. Doses of 50, 125 and 250 mg/kg bw/day were administered for 14 days. At the end of the study, blood was taken from the animals. All the mice were examined macroscopically. Body weight gain was normal except for an increase in body weight in the males given 125 and 250 mg/kg and a reduction in the females given 250 mg/kg. On investigation of organ weights (brain, liver, spleen, lungs, thymus, kidneys, testes), an increase in the absolute and relative liver weights was seen in male mice given 125 and 250 mg/kg and in females given 250 mg/kg. The following haematological parameters were unaffected by bromoform administration: leukocyte, erythrocyte and thrombocyte counts, haemoglobin concentration and haematocrit level. In the males, the fibrinogen value was reduced at the top dose level, and the prothrombin time was reduced at all dose levels. Clinical-chemical parameters [calcium, sodium, chloride, potassium, protein, cholesterol, bilirubin, creatinine, lactate dehydrogenase, serum glutamate-pyruvate transaminase (SGPT), alkaline phosphatase] were normal, except for a decrease in the glucose and urea levels and an increase in the serum glutamate-oxaloacetate transaminase (SGOT) levels in males in the 250 mg/kg dose group; in females, only SGOT levels were raised.

Condie et al. (1983) investigated the subacute oral toxicity of bromoform in male CD1 mice. The chemical was made up in oil and administered at 0.1 mg/30 g body weight for 14 consecutive days. Doses used were 0, 72, 145 and 289 mg/kg body weight. At the end of the study the animals were killed and examined macroscopically. Tissues of the liver and kidneys were examined microscopically. The following parameters were determined in the blood: urea, creatinine and SGPT. In addition, the active transport of p-aminohippuric acid in slices of the kidney cortex was studied as an indicator of the functional ability of the proximal tubules. Only in the highest dose group was the active uptake of p-aminohippuric acid significantly inhibited by about 30%; the SGPT values were likewise increased only in this group. The rest of the clinical-chemical parameters investigated were unchanged. Microscopic examination revealed dose-dependent hyperplasia of the epithelium of the kidney tubules and hypertrophy and degenerative changes in the glomerulae in the medium- and high-dose groups. In the liver, paleness of the centrolobular cytoplasm and inflammation reactions were diagnosed, and there was an increase in the rate of mitosis in the hepatocytes.

Chu et al. (1982 b) administered bromoform in the drinking water of groups of ten male Sprague-Dawley rats (newly weaned) at concentrations of 0, 5, 50 or 500 ppm for 28 days. Emulphor served as a solvent. Both controls comprised ten rats each, receiving either tap water alone or tap water together with the solvent. Water and food intake were checked twice weekly, and the weight of the animals was determined at weekly intervals. Based on the measurements of water intake per animal, the following dose rates were calculated for bromoform: 0.13, 1.5 and 14 mg/rat (~0.65, 7.5, 70 mg/kg) per day. The following blood parameters were determined at the end of the study: sodium, potassium, calcium, organic phosphate, bilirubin, alkaline phosphatase, glutamateoxaloacetate transaminase (GOT), total protein, cholesterol, glucose, uric acid, lactate dehydrogenase, sorbitol dehydrogenase, haemoglobin, erythrocyte count, haematocrit level, differential blood count and platelet count. The cell content of the bone marrow was measured as well as the activity of aniline hydroxylase, aryl hydrocarbon hydroxylase, aminopyrine-demethylase, glutamyl-transpeptidase and ornithine-carbamoyl transferase. The following organs were weighed: brain, liver, spleen, kidney and heart. In addition to macroscopic examination of the animals, the following tissues were examined microscopically: brain, hypophysis, liver, adrenal glands, thyroid gland, epithelial bodies, thymus, trachea, bronchi, thoracic aorta, oesophagus, stomach (cardiac, fundus and pylorus regions), duodenum, pancreas, colon, kidney, spleen, bone marrow, lymph nodes of the mesentery and mediastinum, testes, epididymis, skeletal muscle and heart. Weight gain and nutrient intake were not influenced by administration of the test substance. Symptoms of toxicity were not observed. Clinical-chemical and haematological parameters and also enzyme activities in the liver were not changed on administration of bromoform. No treatment-related pathological changes were found in the organs investigated.

Dykan (1964) carried out a subacute dermal study in rats and guinea-pigs. Doses of 100–200 mg bromoform/kg were applied topically for 10 days. Changes were observed in the following parameters: urinary protein content, creatinine levels in the blood and urine, nitrogen levels in the blood, liver glycogen content and prothrombin time. Moreover, treatment-related damage was diagnosed in the liver and kidneys. Further details on this study are not available (abstract from a Russian paper).

Similarly, Dykan (1965) carried out a subacute inhalation study in rats. The animals were exposed to a bromoform concentration of 2.5 mg/l. Disturbances of protein metabolism and glycogen synthesis in the liver occurred, along with adverse effects on the filtration capacity of the kidneys. Dystrophic changes were also found in the liver and kidneys. Further details are not available (abstract from a Russian paper).

The same author reported on a further subacute inhalation study in rats, which were exposed to 0.25 mg bromoform/l air for 4 hours daily for 2 months. The toxic effects manifested as disturbances in important liver functions (protein synthesis, glycogenesis) and impairment of the filtration capacity of the kidneys. Further details of the study are not available (Dykan, 1965).

7.3 Skin and mucous membrane effects

On repeated application to rabbit skin, bromoform was only slightly irritating. The undiluted solution had only a mild irritant effect on rabbits' eyes. The changes were reversible after 1–2 days (no further details; Torkelson and Rowe, 1981).

7.4 Sensitization

No information available

7.5 Subchronic and chronic toxicity

Groups of 20 male and female Sprague-Dawley rats (newly weaned) received bromoform in the drinking water at concentrations of 0, 5, 50, 500 and 2500 ppm for 90 days. Based on the water intake, the actual quantity of bromoform ingested was calculated as 0.16, 1.5, 14 and 50 mg/rat (corresponding to 0.8, 7.5, 70, 250 mg/kg) per day for males and 0.11, 1.2, 9.6 and 45 mg/rat (corresponding to 0.55, 6.0, 98, 255 mg/kg) per day for females. After 90 days, ten males and ten females from each group were killed. The remaining rats were observed for a further 90 days. All animals were studied macroscopically. The organ weights, biochemical and haematological parameters, and activities of liver enzymes were determined as in the 28-day experiment described above. The same organs were also examined histologically. Deaths during the treatment period included one male from the high-dose group, two females from the 500 ppm group, and one female from the 5 ppm group. During the observation period, one female rat died from each of the 50 ppm, 500 ppm and 2500 ppm groups. All of these animals became emaciated prior to death. Microscopic examination revealed "atrophy of the liver" and extensive sloughing of the cells lining the oesophagus and the entrance to the stomach. Pyelonephritis was seen in one animal in the 500 ppm group (at the end of the observation period). At the highest dose level, food intake in male rats was reduced. There was a trend towards reduced weight-gain in all treatment groups, but this was no longer evident at the end of the 90-day observation period. A treatment-related reduction in lactate dehydrogenase activity was observed in males and females of the 2500 ppm group. This effect remained after the 90-day observation period. Moreover, there were changes in the liver (fatty degeneration and vacuolization, increased thickness of the periportal area) and in the thyroid gland (reduced follicle size and colloid content). No dose-dependency was established for the mild to moderate damage to the liver and thyroid gland, but the effects were increased in the highest dose group. After 90 days of observation, the changes in the liver and thyroid gland were almost reversed. In the highest dose group, a reduction in the number of lymphocytes occurred, an effect which had not been evident at the end of the treatment period. The other dosage groups were not investigated (Chu et al., 1982 a).

## 7.6 Genotoxicity

### 7.6.1 In vitro

Simmon et al. (1977) studied the mutagenic activity of bromoform in the Ames test using strains TA 1535 and TA 100. A metabolising system was not added. The indicator organisms were put in open plates for 8 hous at 37 °C in a 9 l desiccator, exposed to the vapour that arose from 50, 100, 150 and 200 µl of the test substance. Bromoform proved to be a dose-dependent mutagen. Quantities above 100 µl exerted a cytotoxic action on bacteria.

Melnick (1989) has described numerous studies on Ames tests in strains TA 97, TA 98, TA 100, TA 1535 and TA 1537, with and without the addition of S9 from Aroclor-treated Syrian hamster or rat livers. Concentrations of 10-6666 µg/plate were tested. No point-mutagenic action resulted. In a few cases the result was questionable or very weakly positive (TA 100).

Bromoform was mutagenic in mouse lymphocytes (L5178Y), whether or not S9 mix was added. The concentrations tested were 25–300 nl/ml without S9 mix and 2.5–50 nl/ml with S9 mix. The lymphocytes ($6 \times 10^5$/ml) were treated with a medium containing the substance for 4 hours at 37 °C, and were then washed and incubated again for 48 hours at 37 °C. At the end, $3 \times 10^6$ cells from each test concentration were mixed with trifluorothymidine and checked for the number of trifluorothymidine-resistant cells (Melnick, 1989).

In an *in vitro* investigation, Chinese hamster ovary cells were incubated with bromoform at concentrations of 50–1070 µg/ml without added S9 mix, and at concentrations of 160–1600 µg/ml with S9 mix. At each concentration, 100 cells were used. In the studies without S9 mix a weakly positive effect on chromosome aberrations was seen, while in the studies with S9 mix there was no significant increase in the aberration rate (Melnick, 1989).

A further *in vitro* study investigated the possible induction of sister chromatid exchange in Chinese hamster ovary cells after treatment with bromoform. Bromoform was tested at concentrations of 16–290 µg/ml without S9 mix and at 50–968 µg/ml with S9 mix. In the absence of S9 mix there was a weak induction of sister chromatid exchange, while in the presence of S9 mix no significant effect on sister chromatid exchange could be established (Melnick, 1989).

Bromoform increases the sister chromatid exchange rate in human lymphocytes treated *in vitro*. Doses of $1.6 \times 10^{-5}$ to $2 \times 10^{-3}$ M were used. The effect was dose-dependent (Morimoto and Koizumi, 1983).

7.6.2 In vivo

In the Drosophila test, bromoform caused increased lethality in male offspring, indicative of point-mutagenic activity. The male parents received 3000 ppm bromoform in 5% sucrose solution orally for 3 days. In a separate experiment, 1000 ppm in 0.7% saline was administered by injection. In both cases, there was an increased rate of lethality in the male offspring, together with an increased incidence of sterility (Melnick, 1989).

In an *in vivo* study to check for chromosomal aberrations, male B6C3F1 mice (10 animals/dose group) received intraperitoneal injections of bromoform (in corn oil) at concentrations of 200, 400 or 800 mg/kg body weight. In dose-finding studies, 800 mg/kg was reported as the maximum tolerated dose. The animals were killed 36 hours after administration of the chemical, and 6 hours after bromodeoxyuridine administration. The bone marrow was then removed from the femur and 50 cells from each animal were examined. There were no indications of clastogenic activity (Melnick, 1989). In a comparable *in vivo* experiment in mice, the induction of sister chromatid exchange in bone marrow cells was evaluated. The doses used correspond to those in the previous investigation. Results showed an increased rate of sister chromatid exchange (Melnick, 1989).

Male ICR/SJ mice (45–50 g) were treated orally for 4 days with bromoform (in olive oil) at dose levels of 0, 25, 50, 100 and 200 mg/kg

**Table 1.** Study design and results of an investigation into the chronic toxicity of bromoform in mice on intraperitoneal administration [a]

| Dose (mg/kg) | Vehicle | Number of i.p. injections (3 times a week) | Total dose (mg/kg) | Numbers of surviving animals/ no. of animals used originally | Numbers of lung tumours/ mouse [b] | p-value |
|---|---|---|---|---|---|---|
| 0 | Tricaprylin | 24 | 0 | 15/20 | $0.27 \pm 0.15$ | [d] |
| 4 | Tricaprylin | 18 | 72 | 17/20 | $0.53 \pm 0.21$ | 0.335 |
| 48 | Tricaprylin | 23 | 1100 | 15/20 | $1.13 \pm 0.36$ | 0.041 [c] |
| 100 | Tricaprylin | 24 | 2400 | 15/20 | $0.63 \pm 0.21$ | 0.136 |
| Control | | | | | | |
| 1000 | Urethane | 1 | 1000 | 20/20 | $19.6 \pm 2.4$ | [d] |
| | 0.9% saline | 24 | 0 | 47/50 | $0.19 \pm 0.08$ | [d] |

[a] Duration of study: 24 weeks
[b] Average ± standard deviation
[c] Significant difference compared with control
[d] No data

per day. A dose-dependent increase in sister chromatid exchange (up to 9 SCEs per cell) was found in the bone marrow cells of these treated mice (Morimoto and Koizumi, 1983).

Male mice received two intraperitoneal injections of bromoform in corn oil within 24 hours at dose levels of 200, 400 and 800 mg/kg body weight. The animals were killed 24 hours after the second injection, and smears from the bone marrow of the femur were prepared and stained. The incidence of micronuclei was assessed in 1000 polychromatic erythrocytes from each animal. A dose-dependent increase in micronuclei occurred after treatment with bromoform (Melnick, 1989).

On oral administration of radiolabelled bromoform (2.7 mCi/mmol, 1.5 mmol/kg) to male Sprague-Dawley rats (225–275 g), no binding of radioactivity to liver DNA took place. The same authors also carried out an initiation study in male Sprague-Dawley rats (225–275 g). A partial hepatectomy was carried out (two-thirds of the organ) under anaesthesia, 20–22 hours prior to oral dosing (by stomach tube) with 0.8 mmol bromoform/kg (about 200 mg/kg) dissolved in tricaprylin (2 ml/kg). Three days later, 500 ppm sodium phenobarbital was administered in the drinking water of the rats for 47 days. The right lateral lobe of the liver was removed and cut into slices 6 days after the end of the phenobarbital treatment. The slices were examined for γ-glutamyl transpeptidase (γ-GTase) activity. The number of γ-GTase-positive foci containing nine or more nuclei were counted. 2 $cm^2$ of tissue from each animal was scanned for such foci. No increase in the incidence of γ-GTase-positive foci was found in the bromoform-treated rats (Pereira et al., 1982).

## 7.7 Carcinogenicity

Theiss et al. (1977) carried out a 24-week study to assess the carcinogenic activity of bromoform on intraperitoneal administration to male mice of the strain A-ST. The animals were 6–8 weeks old at the start of the study. Before the main experiment, the maximum tolerated dose (MTD) was ascertained, this being the dose that did not cause any deaths amongst groups of five treated mice given six intraperitoneal injections over a period of 2 weeks, with an observation period of 4 weeks. An MTD of 100 mg/kg was estimated for bromoform, and this was the highest dose used in the main experiment. Two further groups received 48 and 4 mg/kg respectively, in each case three times a week by intraperitoneal injection with a maximum of 24 injections. The animals were killed 24 weeks after the first injection, and the number of lung adenomas was counted. The design of the study and its results are detailed in Table 1. Mice of this strain had only a low incidence of lung adenomas after administration of 0.9% saline. In comparison, after administration of urethane (positive control) a strikingly high incidence was seen. With bromoform, a significant increase in the number of lung adenomas per mouse was only found in the middle-dose group compared to the controls, but the number of lung adenomas per mouse was also higher than the controls in the low- and high-dose groups. However, compared to the result with urethane as a positive control, the effect was only slight. The result can therefore only be evaluated as a weak indication of the possible carcinogenic activity of bromoform (Theiss et al., 1977).

Groups of 40 rats of each sex received bromoform in microcapsules with their food for 24 months at concentrations of 40, 1600 and 6500 ppm. Some animals were killed after 6, 12 and 18 months, and the remainder at 24 months. Standard investigations, such as haematology, clinical chemistry, determination of organ weight and macroscopic and microscopic pathology were carried out in each case. In the high- and medium-dose groups, body-weight gain was clearly retarded. In the high-dose group, histopathological effects were seen in the liver (vacuolization and swelling of the hepatocytes, microgranuloma formation, proliferation of the bile duct and cholangiofibrosis). Clinical-chemical investigations revealed a reduction in fatty acids, triglycerides and cholinesterase activity, and an increase in glutamate-pyruvate transaminase and glutamyl transpeptidase activity, correlating with the histopathological findings in the liver. Signs of carcinogenic activity were not identified, but these are only preliminary results and an evaluation of the histopathological findings has not yet been published (Tobe, 1988).

In a further long-term oral study, 50 Fischer rats of each sex received bromoform (in corn oil) by stomach tube at doses of 100 and 200 mg/kg body weight, given for 5 days per week over 103 weeks. The results revealed a reduced final body weight in the males in both dose groups and the females in the high-dose group. With the exception of the males in the high-dose group, the survival rate of the treated rats corresponded with that of the controls. A clearly reduced survival rate was evident in the males of the high-dose group. Non-neoplastic changes found in the males included fatty infiltration of the liver, inflammatory foci, and minimal necrosis, and in the females, fatty infiltration of the liver and inflammatory infiltrations. There was "some evidence" of carcinogenicity in male rats, with two adenomatous polyps and one adenocarcinoma of the intestine in the high-dose group. In female rats there was "clear evidence" of carcinogenicity with six adenomatous polyps and two adenocarcinomas of the intestine in the high-dose group and one adenomatous polyp in the low-dose group (Melnick, 1989).

In a comparable oral long-term study in B6C3F1 mice, 50 animals of each sex received bromoform by stomach tube at dose levels of 50 or 100 mg/kg body weight for 103 weeks. Administration was likewise carried out for 5 days/week. Corn oil was used as the vehicle. The results showed a reduction in body-weight gain by the females in both dose groups compared with controls, but no such effect was seen in the males. A reduced survival rate was also seen in both treated and control females, whilst the males showed a normal survival rate. Non-neoplastic changes found in the females included fatty liver infiltration and follicular hyperplasia of the thyroid gland. There were no conspicuous findings in the males. Neoplastic changes did not occur in either sex. However, it should be noted that infections of the uteri and ovaries occurred in the females, which may have been responsible for the reduced survival rate (Melnick, 1989).

## 7.8 Reproductive toxicity

Ruddick et al. (1980, 1983) investigated the possible teratogenic effect of bromoform. In each case, bromoform was administered by stomach tube to 15 pregnant Sprague-Dawley rats from days 6–15 of pregnancy at dose levels of 50, 100 and 200 mg/kg/day. Fifteen animals served as controls. The rats were killed on the 22nd day of pregnancy. The following parameters were determined in order to study the toxic effects on the mother: weight, haemoglobin concentration, haematocrit level, erythrocyte and leukocyte count and bone marrow cytology. Liver, heart, brain, spleen and kidneys were macroscopically evaluated. The following were examined microscopically: brain, heart, hypophysis, thyroid gland, thymus, lungs, trachea, bronchi, bronchial nodes, liver, kidneys, adrenal glands, spleen, skeletal muscle, peripheral nerves, salivary glands, skin, bone marrow, ovaries, uterus and bladder. A series of clinical-chemical parameters was also determined: sodium, potassium, calcium, inorganic phosphate, bilirubin, alkaline phosphatase, glutamateoxaloacetate transaminase, total protein, cholesterol, glucose, uric acid, lactate dehydrogenase and sorbitol dehydrogenase. Protein, aniline dehydrogenase activity and aminopyrine demethylase activity were determined in liver homogenates. Possible toxic effets on the foetus were evaluated in terms of litter size, foetal weight, deciduomalformation, and visceral and skeletal malformations. The foetuses from the mothers in the high-dose and low-dose groups were examined microscopically (not further defined). Bromoform was not maternally toxic according to all the given parameters. Sternebral aberrations and interparietal deviations were seen in a few foetuses in various litters, and were considered to be dose-related embryotoxic effects. No histological effects in the foetuses were reported.

7.9 Effects on the immune system

Munson et al. (1982) investigated the influence of repeated oral administration to CD1 mice (Charles-River, 7–10 animals/dose) of 50, 125 or 250 mg bromoform/kg (given by stomach tube) on the humoral and cellular immune response. The humoral immune response was investigated in a plaque assay according to Jerne and Nordin (1963) modified according to Cunningham and Szenberg (1968). Estimation of cellular immune response was carried out with the aid of the DTH-response (foot pad assay) based on the method of Lagrange et al. (1973). In both experiments, SRBC (sheep red blood cells) served as the stimulant. The results indicated that the humoral immune response (number of antibody-forming B-lymphocytes in the spleen) was clearly suppressed (ca. 50%) in males in the high-dose group, with a comparable effect on the cellular immune response. The animals treated with bromoform were only about half as strongly stimulated by the SRBC as the corresponding controls. No such effect on the immune system was seen in the males in the remaining dose groups or in any of the treated females.

7.10 Neurotoxicity

No information available.

7.11 Other effects

No information available.

## 8. Experience in humans

Cases of poisoning with bromoform have mainly been observed in children ingesting the chemical. Breathing difficulties, cyanosis, accelerated pulse and unconsciousness are seen. According to the authors, the amount of bromoform swallowed was between 8 drops and 7 g (Lewin and Guillery, 1913).

## 9. Threshold limit values

In the USA a threshold limit value of 5 $mg/m^3$ air has been stated.

## References

ACGIH (American Conference of Governmental Industrial Hygienists)
TLV's, Threshold Limit Values and Biological Exposure Indices for 1988–1989
Cincinnati, Ohio

Ahmed, A.E., Kubic, V.L., Anders, M.W.
Metabolism of haloforms to carbon monoxide, I. In vitro studies
Drug Metab. Dispos., 5, 198–204 (1977)

Anders, M.W., Stevens, J.L., Sprague, R.W., Shaath, Z., Ahmed, A.E.
Metabolism of haloforms to carbon monoxide, II. In vivo studies
Drug Metab. Dispos., 6, 556–560 (1978)

Binz, C.
Zur Umwandlung des Bromoforms im Warmblüter
Arch. Exp. Pathol. Pharmakol., 28, 201–205 (1891)

Bowman, F.J., Borzelleca, J.F., Munson, A.E.
The toxicity of some halomethanes in mice
Toxicol. Appl. Pharmacol., 44, 213–215 (1978)

Chu, I., Secours, V.E., Marino, I., Villeneuve, D.C.
The acute toxicity of four trihalomethanes in male and female rats
Toxicol. Appl. Pharmacol., 52, 351–353 (1980)

Chu, I., Villeneuve, D.C., Secours, V.E., Becking G.C.
Toxicity of trihalomethanes: I. The acute and subacute toxicity of chloroform, bromodichloromethane, chlorodibromomethane and bromoform in rats
J. Environ. Sci. Health, B17 (3), 205–224 (1982 a)

Chu, I., Villeneuve, D.C., Secours, V.E., Becking, G.C.
Trihalomethanes: II. Reversibility of toxicological changes produced by chloroform, bromodichloromethane, chlorodibromomethane and bromoform in rats
J. Environ. Sci. Health, B17 (3), 225–240 (1982 b)

Condie, L.W., Smallwood, C.L., Laurie, R.D.
Comparative renal and hepatotoxicity of halomethanes: Bromodichloromethane, bromoform, chloroform, dibromochloromethane and methylene chloride
Drug Chem. Toxicol., 6 (6), 563–578 (1983)

Cunningham, A.G., Szenberg, A.
Further improvements in the plaquing technique for detecting single antibody forming cells
Immunology, 14, 599–600 (1968)

Dykan, V.A.
Changes in liver and kidney functions due to methylenebromide and bromoform
Chem. Abstr., 60, 8541 d (1964)

Dykan, V.A.
Problems on toxicology, clinical practice and work hygiene in the production of bromine-organic compounds
Chem. Abstr., 63, 15429 g (1965)

Jerne, N.K., Nordin, A.A.
Plaque formation in agar by single antibody producing cells
Science, 140, 405 (1963)

Kutob, S.D., Plaa, G.L.
A procedure for estimating the hepatotoxic potential of certain industrial solvents
Toxicol. Appl. Pharmacol., 4, 354–361 (1962)

Lagrange, P.H., Mackaness, G.B., Müller, T.E.
Influence of dose and route of antigen injection on the immunological induction of T cells
J. Exp. Med., 139, 528–542 (1973)

Lewin, C., Guillery, H.
Die Wirkungen von Arzneimitteln und Giften auf das Auge
August Hirschwald Verlag, Berlin, 45–46 (1913)

Melnick, R.L.
Toxicology and carcinogenesis studies of tribromomethane (bromoform) (CAS No. 75-25-2) in F344/N rats and B6C3F1 mice (gavage studies)
NTP, TR 350. US Dep. Health & Human Serv., Research Triangle Park, NC (1989)

Morimoto, K., Koizumi, A.
Trihalomethanes induce sister chromatid exchange in human lymphocytes in vitro and mouse bone marow cells in vivo
Environ. Res., 32, 72–79 (1983)

Muson, A.E., Sain, L.E., Sanders, V.M., Kauffmann, B.M., White, K.L., Page, D.G., Barns, D.W., Borzelleca, J.F.
Toxicology of organic drinking water contaminants:
Trichloromethane, bromodichloromethane, dibromochloromethane and tribromomethane
Environ. Health Perspect, 46, 117–126 (1982)

Neumüller, O.A. (ed.)
Römpps Chemie-Lexikon
8th ed., p. 522 (1979)
Franckh'sche Verlagshandlung, Stuttgart

Pereira, M.A., Lin, L.H.C., Lipitt, J.M., Herren, S.L.
Trihalomethanes as initiators and promoters of carcinogenesis
Environ. Health Perspect, 46, 151–156 (1982)

Ruddick, J.A., Villeneuve, D.C., Chu, I., Valli, V.E.
Teratogenicity assessment of four trihalomethanes
Teratology, 21, 66 A (1980)

Ruddick, J.A., Villeneuve, D.C., Chu, I.
The teratological assessment of four trihalomethanes in the rat
J. Environ. Sci. Health, B18 (3), 333–349 (1983)

Simmon, V.F., Kauhonen, K., Tardiff, R.G.
Mutagenic activity of chemicals identified in drinking water
In: Progress in genetic toxicology
Scott, D., Bridges, B.A., Sobels, F.H. (eds.)
Elsevier/North Holland Biomedical Press (1977)

Stevens, J.U., Anders, M.W.
Metabolism of haloforms to carbon monoxide
III. Studies on the mechanism of the reaction
Biochem. Pharmacol., 28, 3189–3194 (1979)

Theiss, J.C., Stoner, G.D., Shimkin, M.B., Weisburger, E.K.
Test for carcinogenicity of organic contaminants of United States drinking waters by pulmonary tumor response in strain A mice
Cancer Res., 37, 2717–2720 (1977)

Tobe, M.
Long-term study (24 months) with bromoform in rats (preliminary results)
National Institute of Hygiene Sciences, Tokyo, Japan
(Communication to BG Chemie of 22.12.1988)

Torkelson, T.R., Rowe, V.K.
Halogenated aliphatic hydrocarbons
Patty's Industrial Hygiene and Toxicology
Clayton, G.D., Clayton, F.E. (eds.), 3rd ed., Vol. IIB, 3469–3470.
John Wiley and Sons, New York (1981)

# Diethylcarbamoyl chloride

## 1. Summary and evaluation

Diethylcarbamoyl chloride undergoes rapid hydrolysis to diethylamine in mammals.

The substance is of low acute toxicity ($LD_{50}$, rats oral # 2000 mg/kg). The central nervous system is affected after oral ingestion and the respiratory tract after inhalation, while no systemic effect is evident following a single dermal application. However, locally (skin, eyes), the substance is severely irritating and corrosive. *in vitro* tests using different strains of bacteria, both with and without metabolic activation, show a weak mutagenic effect, whilst the substance induces no DNA repair in isolated rat hepatocytes. The substance acts as a carcinogen on mouse skin if repeatedly applied epicutaneously in combination with a promoter (phorbol myristate acetate).

On the basis of its acylating property, diethylcarbamoyl chloride may possess carcinogenic potential.

Since 1978, diethylcarbamoyl chloride has been in section III B of the German list of TLV's (DFG, 1978).

## 2. Name of substance

| | | |
|---|---|---|
| 2.1 | Usual name | Diethylcarbamoyl chloride |
| 2.2 | IUPAC-name | N,N-Diethylcarbamoyl chloride |
| 2.3 | CAS-No. | 88-10-8 |

## 3. Synonyms, common and trade names

Diethylcarbamic acid chloride
Diethylcarbamoylchlorid
Diethylcarbamyl chloride
Diethylcarbamidsäurechlorid

## 4. Structural and molecular formulae

4.1 Structural formula

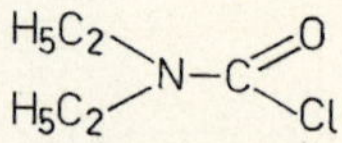

4.2 Molecular formula $C_5H_{10}ClNO$

## 5. Physical and chemical properties

| | | |
|---|---|---|
| 5.1 | Molecular mass, g/mol | 135.59 |
| 5.2 | Melting point, °C | –32 (BASF, 1988) |
| 5.3 | Boiling point, °C | 186 (BASF, 1988) |
| 5.4 | Vapour pressure, hPa | 1 (at 20 °C) (BASF, 1988)<br>9 (at 50 °C) (BASF, 1988) |
| 5.5 | Density, $g/cm^3$ | 1.073 at 20 °C (BASF, 1988) |
| 5.6 | Solubility in water | Hydrolyses (BASF, 1988) |
| 5.7 | Solubility in organic solvents | No information available |
| 5.8 | Solubility in fat | No information available |
| 5.9 | pH-value | – |
| 5.10 | Conversion factor | 1 ppm ≅ 5.626 $mg/m^3$<br>1 $mg/m^3$ ≅ 0.178 ppm<br>(at 25 °C and 1013 hPa)<br>(BASF, 1988) |

## 6. Uses

Versatile intermediate, especially for use in the production of pesticides (Paetsch, 1986; Sax, 1979).

## 7. Experimental results

7.1 Toxicokinetics and metabolism

Wistar rats (initial weight 280 g, sex and group size not given) inhaled increasing concentrations (2.5–250 ppm) of diethylcarbamoyl chloride (DECC) over a period of 15 minutes (no detailed information given). Blood diethylamine levels were determined on the spectrophotometer after the animals were killed. The results showed rapid hydrolysis of the chemical to diethylamine. From the relationship between the atmospheric concentration of DECC and the blood level of diethylamine, extensive absorption of DECC from the inhaled air is thought to occur (Anger et al., 1981).

7.2 Acute and subacute toxicity

Single doses of 1470, 1780, 2150, 2610, 3160 and 4640 mg DECC/kg body weight were administered in olive oil by stomach tube to groups of five male and five female fasted Sprague-Dawley rats (average weights 225 and 168 g respectively, housed under standard conditions). The observation period was 14 days. Mortality, symptoms of toxicity and the findings at autopsy (for the rats which died during the experiment and those killed at the end of the study) were reported, along with the median lethal dose. An approximate $LD_{50}$ of 2000 mg DECC/kg body weight was calculated for both sexes. Depending on the dose administered, death occurred within 1 to 25 hours. The observed symptoms indicate an effect on the central nervous system (atonia, narcosis). The rats which died during the experiment showed dilation of the heart with congestive hyperaemia and an atonal gastro-intestinal tract. No effects were seen in the animals killed at the end of the observation period (BASF, 1979).

To study the systemic toxicity of DECC from a single dermal application, 200 mg DECC/kg body weight were applied to the shaved backs (ca. 50 $cm^2$) of groups of five male and five female rabbits (white Viennese, average weight 1.4 and 2.3 kg respectively, housed under standard conditions). The application site was covered with aluminium foil which was secured with adhesive tape. The dressing was removed 24 hours after application, and the remaining substance washed off with water or a water/polyethylene glycol-400 mixture. Over an observation period of 8 days, the rabbits were assessed for systemic toxicity, local skin changes and, following autopsy, effects on the internal organs. All animals tolerated acute dermal treatment without systemic symptoms, and no deaths occurred. Primary irritation was evident 24 hours after application, which cleared within 8 days. Autopsy of the animals killed at the end of the observation period revealed no treatment-related effects on the internal organs. The $LD_{50}$ value on acute dermal application is thus more than 200 mg DECC/kg body weight (BASF, 1979).

An intraperitoneal $LD_{50}$ value of 750 mg DECC/kg body weight has been reported (no further details; Sax, 1979).

Six to 12 rats were exposed to a vapour-enriched atmosphere at 20 °C for up to 8 hours. Deaths, clinical findings and the results of autopsies were reported. Three out of six animals died after a 3-hour exposure, and after 8 hours, five of the six were dead. Symptoms observed included dyspnoea and severe irritation of the mucous membranes. At autopsy, oedema, emphysema and congestion of the lungs were seen, as well as bloody serous encrusting of the snouts (BASF, 1970).

### 7.3 Skin and mucous membrane effects

Undiluted DECC was applied as a patch test to the backs of rabbits (sex and number not given) for 1, 5 or 15 minutes or 20 hours. The skin was evaluated for local effects 24 hours and 8 days after application. The effects seen 24 hours after application increased with the exposure time, from slight to moderate or severe reddening to oedema formation. After 8 days, similar but somewhat diminished effects were seen, accompanied by marked hyperkeratosis (BASF, 1970).

DECC (0.5 ml) was tested for irritant effects in rabbits' eyes. After 1 hour, severe irritation of the conjunctiva and slight oedema formation were seen. The cornea was slightly clouded. Evaluation after 24 hours showed comparable effects, except that the cornea was more severely clouded. The conjunctiva and cornea appeared normal 8 days after application (BASF, 1970).

### 7.4 Sensitization

No information available.

### 7.5 Subchronic and chronic toxicity

No information available.

### 7.6 Genotoxicity

#### 7.6.1 In vitro

Nelson (1977) cited unpublished results from Mukai, according to which DECC was mutagenic in *Salmonella typhimurium* (no further details) and *Escherichia coli* WP2 and WP2S (10.4 mg/plate) without metabolic activation.

Oesch (1978) reported that DECC had a very weak mutagenic effect in the bacterial strains TA 1535 and TA 100 in the Salmonella/microsome test at concentrations of 2400 µl/plate and above (test concentration 24–7200 µl/plate), while in strains TA 1537 and TA 98 no mutagenic activity was seen. The addition of S9 mix (liver homogenate from Aroclor pre-treated Sprague-Dawley rats) decreased the mutagenic activity of DECC.

According to Probst et al. (1981) the highest non-toxic concentration of DECC (500 nmol/ml) does not induce DNA repair (unscheduled DNA synthesis) in a primary culture of hepatocytes from male Fischer-344 rats.

Segal et al. (1982) showed that DECC reacts with deoxyguanine *in vitro* to form the $O^6$-acyl derivative, 6-diethylcarbamyloxy-2'-deoxyguanosine, which was considered by the authors to be an essential trigger of mutagenic activity.

7.6.2 In Vivo

No information available

7.7 Carcinogenicity

As part of a study on structure-activity relationships in carcinogenicity, van Duuren (1980, 1987) reported a long-term study with DECC on 30 female ICR/Ha Swiss mice. The results are summarised in Table 1. On the basis of its acylating property, DECC may possess cacinogenic potential. The design of the study and the reporting and evaluation of the results, however, were insufficiently documented.

7.8 Reproductive toxicity

No information available

7.9 Effects on the immune system

No information available

7.10 Neurotoxicity

No information available

7.11 Other effects

No information available

## 8. Experience in humans

The lymphocytes of ten workers (100 cells per individual) who had been exposed to DECC (amongst other chemicals) for between 4 and 17 years were examined for chromosomal effects, including gaps, bridges, fragmentation, dicentric rings, translocations and deletions. Ten people of a similar age who had had no contact with DECC were used as controls. There was no significant difference between the two groups (Fleig and Thiess, 1978).

**Table 1.** Carcinogenic activity of DECC on mouse skin

| | | | |
|---|---|---|---|
| Strain | ICR/Ha | ICR/Ha | ICR/Ha |
| Sex | ♀ | ♀ | ♀ |
| Number/group | 30 | 30 | 30 |
| Treatment and dose[a] | DECC, 15 mg 1 x followed by PMA[b], 5 µg 3 x per week | PMA[b], 5 µg 3 x per week | DECC, 5mg 3 x per week subcutaneous |
| Duration of study (days) | 498 | 498 | 504 |
| Median survival time (days) | >498 | >498 | >504 |
| Occurrence of first tumour (day of study) | 254 | 449 | 273 |
| Mice with tumours at the site of application | | | |
| Papillomas | 9 | 3 | 3 |
| of which carcinomas | 2 | 1 | 1[c] |

[a] Application of the substance to the dorsal skin in 0.2 ml acetone
[b] PMA: Phorbol myristate acetate
[c] Squamous carcinoma of the skin with metastases in the lungs

## 9. Threshold limit values

Since 1978, DECC has been in section III B of the German list of maximum acceptable workplace concentrations (DFG, 1978).

## References

Anger, J.P., Corbel, J.C., Paulet, G.
Determination of low levels of diethylcarbamoylchloride in air. First results after inhalation in rats.
Toxicol. Eur. Res., 3, 223–228 (1981)

BASF AG, Gewerbehygienisches-Pharmakologisches Institut
Unpublished report of 14. 8. 1970

BASF AG, Gewerbehygiene und Toxikologie
Bericht über die Prüfung der akuten dermalen Toxizität von „Diäthylcarbaminsäurechlorid" an der Rückenhaut weißer Kaninchen.
Unpublished report of 20. 7. 1979

BASF AG
Communication of 27. 12. 1988

DFG (Deutsche Forschungsgemeinschaft)
Maximum concentrations at the workplace and biological tolerance values for working materials 1978 report no. XIV
Commission for the investigation of health hazards of chemical compounds in the work area
Verlag Chemie, Weinheim (1978)

Duuren van, B.L.
Prediction of carcinogenicity based on structure, chemical reactivity and possible metabolic pathways
J. Environ. Pathol. Toxicol., 3, 11–34 (1980)

Duuren van, B.L., Melchionne, S., Seidman, I.
Carcinogenicity of acylating agents: Chronic bioassays in mice and structure-activity relationships (SARC)
J. Am. Coll. Toxicol., 6, 479–487 (1987)

Fleig, J., Theiss, A.M.
Chromosome investigations of persons exposed to dimethylcarbamoyl chloride and diethylcarbamoyl chloride
Mutat. Res., 53, 188 (1978)

Nelson, N.
The carcinogenicity of chloro ethers and related compounds: A brief note
Cold Spring Harbor Conf. Cell Prolif., 4, 115–118 (1977)

Oesch, F.
Ames-test for diethylcarbamyl chloride and dimethylcarbamyl chloride
Pharmacological institute of the University of Mainz
Commissioned by BASF AG, report of 10. 6. 1978

Paetsch, J.
Carbamates and carbamoyl chlorides
Ullmann's encyclopedia of industrial chemistry
Vol. A5, p. 53–56
VCH Verlagsgesellschaft, Weinheim (1986)

Probst, G.S., McMahont, R.E., Hill, L.E., Thompson, C.Z., Epp, J.K., Neal, S.B.
Chemically-induced unscheduled DNA syntheses in primary rat hepatocyte cultures: A comparison with bacterial mutagenicity using 218 compounds
Environ. Mutagen., 3, 11–32 (1981)

Sax, N.J. (ed.)
Dangerous properties of industrial materials
5th ed., p. 573
van Nostrand Reinhold Co., New York (1979)

Segal A., Solomon, J.J., Maté, U., van Duuren, B.L.
Formation of 6-dimethylcarbamyloxy-dGuo, 6-dimethylamino-dGuo and 4-dimethylamino-dThd following in vitro reaction of dimethylcarbamyl chloride with calf thymus DNA, and 6-diethylcarbamyloxy-dGuo following in vitro reaction of diethylcarbamyl chloride with calf thymus DNA
Chem. Biol. Interact., 40, 209–231 (1982)

# o-Chlorobenzotrifluoride

## 1. Summary and assessment

o-Chlorobenzotrifluoride appears to be of low acute toxicity ($LD_{50}$, rat oral, 1600–2000 and 2900 mg/kg). The toxic symptoms (impairment of motor function and breathing, narcosis and non-specific symptoms) are due to an effect on the central nervous system. All symptoms are reversible in the surviving animals after 6 days. Anatomical/pathological investigation of the animals which died during the study reveals effects on the lungs, liver, kidneys and adrenal glands, as well as irritant effects on the pancreas and on the epithelium of the gut. The surviving animals investigated at the end of the observation period show no changes.

In rabbits, the chemical causes irritation to the skin but not to the eyes.

In mutagenicity tests *in vitro*, o-chlorobenzotrifluoride does not induce point mutations or chromosome aberrations, and does not interact with DNA. Further mutagenicity investigations, including *in vivo* studies, are currently being carried out for the US Department of Health and Human Services.

From industrial experience it is known that vapour inhalation and skin absorption may affect the central nervous system, with possible narcosis.

## 2. Name of substance

| | | |
|---|---|---|
| 2.1 | Usual name | o-Chlorobenzotrifluoride |
| 2.2 | IUPAC-name | 2-Chloro-α,α,α-trifluorotoluene |
| 2.3 | CAS-No. | 88-16-4 |

## 3. Synonyms, common and trade names

2-Chloro-1-trifluoro-
methylbenzene
2-Chlorobenzotrifluoride

## 4. Structural and molecular formulae

4.1 Structural formula

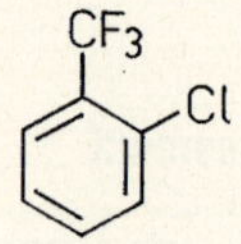


4.2 Molecular formula $C_7H_4ClF_3$

## 5. Physical and chemical properties

| | | |
|---|---|---|
| 5.1 | Molecular mass, g/mol | 180.56 |
| 5.2 | Melting point, °C | -7 (Hoechst, 1985a) |
| 5.3 | Boiling point, °C | 152 (Hoechst, 1985a) |
| 5.4 | Vapour pressure, hPa | 5.32 (at 20 °C) (Hoechst, 1985a)<br>6.65 (at 25 °C) (Hoechst, 1985a) |
| 5.5 | Density, $g/cm^3$ | 1.367 (at 20 °C) (Hoechst, 1985a) |
| 5.6 | Solubility in water | Very slight (Hoechst, 1985a) |
| 5.7 | Solubility in organic solvents | Very soluble (Hoechst, 1985a) |
| 5.8 | Solubility in fat | Dissolves well (Hoechst, 1985a) |
| 5.9 | pH-value | - |
| 5.10 | Conversion factor | 1 ppm $\hat{=}$ 7.4 $mg/m^3$<br>1 $mg/m^3$ $\hat{=}$ 0.14 ppm<br>(at 25 °C and 1013 hPa) |

## 6. Uses

Intermediate for pesticides and dyestuffs (Ciba-Geigy, 1975; Hoechst, 1985a).

## 7. Experimental results

7.1 Toxicokinetics and metabolism

No information available.

7.2 Acute and subacute toxicity

o-Chlorobenzotrifluoride is of low acute toxicity in rats, with an oral $LD_{50}$ of 1600 to 2000 mg/kg body weight in males and 2900 mg/kg body weight in females. In addition to nonspecific symptoms, the toxic effects included impairment of motor function and breathing, blood-stained secretions from the eyes and nose, mydriasis, lack of reflexes (narcosis) and diarrhoea. All symptoms were reversed 6 days after exposure. Macroscopic examination of the dead animals revealed changes to the lungs, liver, kidneys and adrenal glands, as well as reddening of the pancreas and the intestinal lining. Blood was detected in the urine. The surviving animals were free from macroscopically visible changes at the end of the study (Hoechst, 1985c).

7.3 Skin and mucous membrane effects

Neat o-chlorobenzotrifluoride (0.5 ml) was applied semiocclusively to the dorsal skin of 3 New Zealand albino rabbits. The exposure time was 4 hours, after which any remaining test substance was removed. The results were evaluated 30 to 60 minutes after removal of the patch, and then at 24, 48 and 72 hours. As some symptoms were still visible after 72 hours, additional evaluations were made after 7 and 14 days. Clear, localized or moderate erythema and very slight to clear, localized oedema were evident at the application site up to 72 hours after removal of the patch. After 7 days, only barely perceptible to clear, localized erythema was observed. The skin was free from erythema and oedema after 14 days. The treated skin of all animals was dry, chapped and flaky after 7 and 14 days. These findings indicate that the substance is a skin irritant in rabbits (Hoechst, 1985b).

o-Chlorobenzotrifluoride (0.1 ml) was instilled into the conjunctival sac of the left eye of each of 3 New Zealand albino rabbits. The untreated right eye served as a control in each case. The treated eyes were rinsed out thoroughly with physiological saline 24 hours after instillation, and at all subsequent examinations when the eyes were still producing secretions or when a corneal investigation with fluorescein sodium solution took place. The eyes were examined 1, 24, 48, and 72 hours after instillation of the test substance.The cornea was inspected for damage under UV light after instillation of one drop of 0.01% fluorescein sodium solution at 24 and 72 hours. Clear hyperaemia of the blood vessels of the conjunctiva was seen in one animal 1 hour after administration. No further signs of irritation were present 24 hours after application. The substance was not irritating to the mucous membranes of the eyes of rabbits (Hoechst, 1985a)

7.4 Sensitization

No information available.

## 7.5 Subchronic and chronic toxicity

No information available.

## 7.6 Genotoxicity

### 7.6.1 In vitro

o-Chlorobenzotrifluoride was tested for point-mutagenic effects in the Salmonella/microsome test in strains TA 98, TA 100, TA 1535, TA 1537 and TA 1538. The study was carried out with and without metabolic activation. The concentrations used were 50, 100 and 500 µg/plate. o-Chlorobenzotrifluoride did not induce point mutations in any of the 5 strains, whether or not S9-mix was added (Mazza et al., 1986).

The substance was tested for point-mutagenic effects in a further study in *Salmonella typhimurium* (strains TA 98, TA 100, TA 1535, TA 1537 and TA 1538) and in *Escherichia coli* strain WP2. The study was carried out with and without metabolic activation. The concentrations tested were 10, 33.3, 100, 333.3, 1000 and 5000 µg/plate. The results showed that o-chlorobenzotrifluoride had no point-mutagenic effect in the 5 Salmonella strains or in *Escherichia coli,* whether or not S9-mix was added (CCR, 1988a).

o-Chlorobenzotrifluoride was tested for its ability to induce chromosomal aberrations in Chinese hamster V79 cells in vitro. The cell cultures were incubated with the following doses for 4 hours: 5, 25 and 65 µg/ml without S9-mix; 5, 25, 50 and 100 µg/ml with S9-mix. The cultures were processed 7, 18 or 28 hours after addition of the test substance and 100 metaphases per culture were screened for structural chromosomal aberrations. The results showed that there was no indication of chromosomal aberrations on treatment of the cultures with the specified concentrations (CCR, 1988b).

The possible effects of o-chlorobenzotrifluoride on DNA were studied in *Bacillus subtilis* (strains PB 1652 and PB 1791) by the soft agar method (standard protocol). Sterile paper discs (9 mm diameter), impregnated with 30 µl of the test substance, were placed in the middle of agar plates on which the test strains were established. After incubation for 24 hours at 37 °C, the zones of growth inhibition around the discs were measured. o-Chlorobenzotrifluoride did not induce DNA damage (Mazza et al., 1986).

o-Chlorobenzotrifluoride was further tested in *Saccharomyces cerevisiae* (strain 6117) with and without the addition of S9-mix, at a concentration of 2000 µg/ml. There were no indications of crossing-over or of gene conversion (Mazza et al., 1986).

7.6.2 In vivo
No information available.

7.7 Carcinogenicity
No information available.

7.8 Reproductive toxicity
No information available.

7.9 Effects on the immune system
No information available.

7.10 Neurotoxicity
See chapter 7.2.

7.11 Other effects
No information available.

## 8. Experience in humans

From industrial experience, possible inhalation of vapour and absorptive uptake through the skin must be assumed, with possible damage to the nervous system and a potential narcotic effect. There are no epidemiological studies available (Ciba-Geigy, 1975).

## 9. Threshold limit values

No information available.

## References

CCR (Cytotest Cell Research GmbH & Co KG)
*Salmonella typhimurium* and *Escherichia coli* reverse mutation assay with o-chlorbenzotrifluoride
Project 115716 (1988a)
Commissioned by BG Chemie

CCR (Cytotest Cell Research GmbH & Co KG)
Chromosome aberration assay in Chinese hamster V 79 cells in vitro with o-chlorbenzotrifluoride
Project 115727 (1988b)
Commissioned by BG Chemie

Ciba-Geigy
Chemical data card No. 294 (1975)

Hoechst AG, Pharma Forschung Toxikologie
o-Chlorbenzotrifluorid – Prüfung auf Augenreizung am Kaninchen
Unpublished report No. 85.1068 (1985a)

Hoechst AG, Pharma Forschung Toxikologie
o-Chlorbenzotrifluorid – Prüfung auf Hautreizung am Kaninchen
Unpublished report No. 85.1122 (1985b)

Hoechst AG, Pharma Forschung Toxikologie
o-Chlorbenzotrifluorid – Prüfung der akuten oralen Toxizität an der männlichen und weiblichen Wistar-Ratte
Unpublished report No. 85.1134 (1985c)

Mazza, G., Dacarro, C., Bonferoni, C., Bonferoni, B.
Studies on the mutagenic activity of benzotrifluoride and 12 derivatives in microbial short-term assays
Farmaco (Prak.), 41, 215–225 (1986)

# Chloro acetic acid methyl ester

## 1. Summary and assessment

Chloroacetatic acid methyl ester is toxic after a single oral or dermal application ($LD_{50}$, rats oral, 107–140 mg/kg, rats dermal 136–470 mg/kg, rabbits dermal 318 mg/kg). Both routes of administration produce the following symptoms: disturbances to balance, squatting, lying on stomach, diarrhoea, spasmodic respiration or difficulty in breathing, together with poor general condition. Comparable symptoms also appear after intraperitoneal injection (mouse i.p. $LD_{50}$ 200–460 mg/kg) and vapour inhalation. With inhalation exposure ($LC_{50}$ >210<315 ppm), marked irritation of the respiratory tract and eyes is also observed.

In sub-acute studies involving repeated inhalation exposure (concentrations of 10, 33 or 100 ppm), the highest concentration impairs breathing and movement, and causes irritation. Body weight gain and food and water intake are also affected. The relative lung weight is increased. Similar effects, though less pronounced, have been observed in the 33 ppm group, predominantly amongst the males. No such effects have been detected in the 10 ppm group.

Experiments on the local irritant action on rabbit skin reveal a corrosive effect. Chloroacetic acid methyl ester is absorbed through the skin (0.5 ml undiluted substance/rabbit caused death). Tests on the irritant effect on the eye indicate damage to the cornea and iris, in addition to the marked signs of inflammation of the conjunctivae. In man, delayed conjunctivitis has been detected due to the effect of vapour.

Test results in the Salmonella/microsome test using five different strains of bacteria, as well as Escherichia coli (WP2 uvrA), with and without a metabolising system (S9 mix from rat liver homogenate) show no detectable mutagenic effect of the substance. In the mouse micronucleous test, no induction of micronuclei has been detected.

## 2. Name of substance

| | | |
|---|---|---|
| 2.1 | Usual name | Chloroacetic acid methyl ester |
| 2.2 | IUPAC-name | Chloroacetic acid methyl ester |
| 2.3 | CAS-No. | 96-34-4 |

## 3. Synonyms, common and trade names

Methylchloroacetate
Methylmonochloroacetate
Chloressigsäuremethylester

## 4. Structural and molecular formulae

4.1 Structural formula

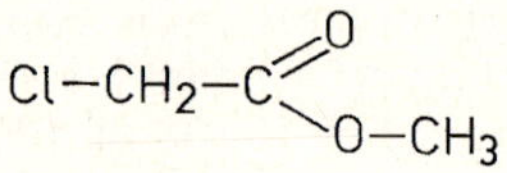

4.2 Molecular formula $C_3H_5ClO_2$

## 5. Physical and chemical properties

| | | |
|---|---|---|
| 5.1 | Molecular mass, g/mol | 108.52 |
| 5.2 | Melting point, °C | -32.12 (Sandmeyer, 1981) |
| 5.3 | Boiling point, °C | 129.8 (Weast, 1982) |
| 5.4 | Vapour pressure, hPa | 3.7 (at 10 °C) (Hoechst, 1986)<br>6.9 (at 20 °C)<br>42.6 (at 50 °C) (Hoechst, 1986) |
| 5.5 | Density, $g/cm^3$ | 1.2337 (at 20 °C) (Sandmeyer, 1981) |
| 5.6 | Solubility in water | 2.8 g/l (at 20 °C) |
| 5.7 | Solubility in organic solvents | good in alcohol, ether, acetone, benzene |
| 5.8 | Solubility in fat | no information available |
| 5.9 | pH-value | 4.6 (Hoechst, 1988) |
| 5.10 | Conversion factor | 1 ppm $\hat{=}$ 4.43 $mg/m^3$<br>1 $mg/m^3$ $\hat{=}$ 0.23 ppm<br>(at 25 °C and 1013 hPa). |

## 6. Uses

Solvent and intermediate in organic synthesis (Windholz, 1983).

## 7. Experimental results

7.1 Toxicokinetics and metabolism
No information available.

7.2 Acute and subacute toxicity

Oral $LD_{50}$ values of 107 mg/kg body weight for the female rat (Hoechst, 1979) and 140 mg/kg body weight for male and female rats (BASF, 1981) have been reported.

On acute dermal administration, the $LD_{50}$ for the rat (sex not given) is about 470 mg/kg body weight (BASF, 1981). A further investigation gave a value of 136 mg/kg body weight in female Wistar rats, and 318 mg/kg body weight in female rabbits (Hoechst, 1979). On dermal application (occlusive, 25–50% or undiluted), skin erythema and oedema formation with subsequent necrosis and partial sloughing of the skin were seen. Those animals that died did so within 24 hours. Autopsy revealed reddening of the small intestine with expansion of the blood vessels and dark-brown coloured and severely vascularized liver, spleen and kidneys.

The $LD_{50}$ value after intraperitoneal injection is between 200 and 460 mg/kg body weight in mice of both sexes (BASF, 1981).

The $LC_{50}$ after acute inhalation exposure for 4 hours was determined as being between 200 and 315 ppm in rats of both sexes. The symptoms predominantly show an effect on the central nervous system (disturbance of balance, squatting, prostration) and on respiration (spasmodic breathing and shortness of breath; Hoechst, 1988a).

In inhalation-risk tests (exposure times of 3, 10, 30 and 50 minutes) the rats died after exposures of 10 minutes and above. In addition to the CNS symptoms (disturbance of balance, squatting, prostration and narcotic effects), symptoms or irritation of the respiratory system and eyes occurred (BASF, 1981).

Groups of 4–5 female rats (strain no given) were exposed to chloroacetic acid methyl ester (purity >95%) by inhalation in a 160 l closed exposure chamber (air flow 15–25 l/minute). Concentrations, inhalation times and mortality are shown in the following table:

| Concentration (ppm) calculated/measured | | Exposure time in hours | Number of dead/ exposed animals |
|---|---|---|---|
| 1000 | 920 | 4.0 | 5/5 |
| 1000 | – | 2.0 | 4/5 |
| 1000 | – | 1.0 | 2/4 |
| 500 | 400 | 4.0 | 5/5 |
| 500 | – | 2.0 | 0/4 |
| 250 | – | 7.0 | 1/5 |
| 250 | – | 4.0 | 0/4 |
| 100 | 81 | 7.0 | 0/4 |

– Not measured.

The rats died a few days after exposure. At autopsy, pneumonia was the predominant effect seen. Chloroacetic acid methyl ester is severely irritating to the respiratory system at concentrations of 250–1000 ppm. At 100 ppm, only a slight irritant effect was seen (Torkelson et al., 1971).

Under the same experimental protocol, two groups of rabbits (number, strain and sex not given) were exposed to chloroacetic acid methyl ester at 100 and 50 ppm for 4 or 7 hours. The animals exhibited irritation of the conjunctiva and cornea at 100 ppm, but not at 50 ppm. The observed irritation was reversible. Staining of the cornea with fluorescein 1 week after exposure showed no corneal damage. All animals survived and there was no weight loss (Torkelson et al., 1971).

In a subacute inhalation study, ten male and ten female Wistar rats (ca. 45 days old, weight 144–161 g) were exposed 20 times in total to chloroacetic acid methyl ester for 6 hours/day, 5 days a week for 4 weeks. At the end of the study, blood was taken from five males and five females for analysis. The animals were dissected, and examined macroscopically and microscopically. The remaining five males and females per dose group served as the recovery group (duration 14 days) and were similarly examined. Results showed eye irritation in the 10 ppm group on the first day of the study. The animals in the 33 ppm group exhibited eye irritation, sneezing and increased frequency of cleaning during exposure. Symptoms were not observed prior to exposure or on the exposure-free days. None of the experimental animals in the 10 and 33 ppm groups showed clinical symptoms during the recovery period. The animals in the 100 ppm group showed eye irritation, sneezing, squatting behaviour, increased frequency of cleaning, irregular breathing, unco-ordinated movement, retracted flanks, reduced activity and ruffled fur. The symptoms were occasionally still present on the following day before exposure, and could still be observed in this dose group during the recovery period, up to day 35 (1 week after the last exposure). No treatment-related effects were seen on the central nervous system, eyes, teeth or mucous membranes of the mouth. Animals in the 100 ppm group showed a clear impairment of body weight gain, although this was partially reversible in the males and completely reversible in the females. Weight gain was also slightly retarded in the males of the 33 ppm group. Animals in the 100 ppm group had reduced food intake and increased drinking water requirements. Haematological, clinical-chemical and urinary investigations gave no indications of toxic damage in the experimental animals. Exposure to 100 ppm chloroacetic acid methyl ester led to a clear increase in relative lung weight. Autopsy of the animals revealed no conspicuous treatment-related macroscopic changes, and microscopic examination of the organ tissues gave no indication of damage. The authors assumed a no effect level for the systemic toxic effects of 33 ppm for the females and 100 ppm for the males (Hoechst, 1988b).

### 7.3 Skin and mucous membrane effects

The test for skin irritation according to FDA guidelines (0.5 ml undiluted product) caused the death of all rabbits within 24 hours. Application of 125 mg/kg body weight (occlusive, 24 hours) produced severe irritant or corrosive effects on the skin (redness, oedema, incrustation; Hoechst, 1979).

The same effects were observed in a further test protocol (BASF-test, 20 hours; Draize-test, 24 hours). Necrosis was seen within 1 hour of exposure (BASF, 1981).

In two studies, the undiluted product caused severe eye irritation. Irreversible damage to the cornea (vascularisation, corneal detachment, scars) and inflammation of the iris was observed (BASF, 1981; Hoechst, 1979).

### 7.4 Sensitization

No information available.

### 7.5 Subschronic and chronic toxicity

No information available.

### 7.6 Genotoxicity

#### 7.6.1 In vitro

Chloroacetic acid methyl ester was tested for mutagenic activity in the Ames test on the bacterial strains TA 100, TA 1535, TA 1537, TA 1538 and TA 98 of *Salmonella typhimurium* and in *Escherichia coli* WP2uvrA, with and without the addition of a metabolic activation system (S9 mix from liver homogenates of Aroclor 1254 pre-treated rats). The product was bacteriotoxic from 2500 µg/plate. Mutagenicity testing was carried out with doses of 4–5000 µg/plate. At the concentrations tested, the substance did not lead to an increase in revertants, either in the presence or absence of a metabolic activation system (Hoechst, 1983).

#### 7.6.2 In vivo

A micronucleus test was carried out with chloroacetic acid methyl ester. The chemical was administered by stomach tube to male and female NMRI-mice (7 weeks old, weight 21–33 g), at the maximum tolerated dose of 300 mg/kg body weight. Five animals of each sex were killed 24, 48 and 72 hours after administration and the erythrocytes appropriately treated. No induction of micronuclei resulted. The ratio of polychromatic to normochromatic erythrocytes was likewise not adversely affected by the treatment (Hoechst, 1988c).

### 7.7 Carcinogenicity

No information available.

### 7.8 Reproductive toxicity

No information available.

### 7.9 Effects on the immune system

No information available.

### 7.10 Neurotoxicity

No information available.

### 7.11 Other effects

No information available.

## 8. Experience in humans

Industrial experience shows that the chemical causes corneal irritation in humans, which is a delayed effect. Further details were not given (Torkelson et al., 1971).

## 9. Threshold limit values

No information available.

## References

BASF AG, Gewerbehygiene und Toxikologie
Unpublished report of 6. 8. 1981

Hoechst AG, Pharma Forschung Toxikologie
Unpublished reports Nos. 139/79, 140/79, 141/79 and 142/79 (1979)

Hoechst AG, Pharma Forschung Toxikologie
Monochloroacetic acid methyl ester
Study of the mutagenic potential in strains of *Salmonella thyphimurium* (Ames Test) and *Escherichia coli*
Unpublished report-Nr. 83.0084 (1983)

Hoechst AG, Pharma Forschung Toxikologie
Communication to BG Chemie (1986)

Hoechst AG, Pharma Forschung Toxikologie
Monochloroacetic acid methyl ester – Inhalation of a mixed stream in male and female SPF-Wistar rats ($LC_{50}$)
Hoechst AG, No. 87.0561 (1988a)
commissioned by BG Chemie

Hoechst AG, Pharma Forschung Toxikologie
Chloroacetic acid methyl ester – Subacute inhalation in SPF-Wistar rats
Hoechst AG, No. 87.0562 (1988b)
commissioned by BG Chemie

Hoechst AG, Pharma Forschung Toxikologie
Monochloroacetic acid methyl ester – Micronucleus test in male and female mice after oral administration
Unpublished report, No.88.1329 (1988c)

Sandmeyer, E.E., Kirwin, C.J.
Esters
Clayton, G.D., Clayton, F.E. (eds.)
Patty's Industrial Hygiene and Toxicology
3rd ed., p. 2384–2391
John Wiley & Sons, New York, 1981

Torkelson, T.R., Kary, C.D., Chenoweth, M.B., Larsen, E.R.
Single exposure of rats to the vapors of trace substances in methoxyflurane
Toxicol. Appl. Pharmacol., 19, 1–9 (1971)

Weast, R.C. (ed.)
CRC-Handbook of Chemistry and Physics
62nd ed., C-227
CRC-Press, Boca Raton, Florida, 1981/82

Windholz, M. (ed.)
The Merck Index, 10th ed., p. 866
Merck and Co., Rahway, N.J., 1983

# m-Chlorobenzotrifluoride

## 1. Summary and assessment

On acute oral administration, m-chlorobenzotrifluoride has been shown to be very slightly toxic, with an $LD_{50}$ value greater than 5000 mg/kg body weight. The symptoms are essentially due to an effect on the central nervous system (impairment of motor function and breathing, confusion and watering of the eyes), and are reversed after 5–6 days of administration. No adverse effect on body weight is observed.

The chemical is not irritating to the skin or mucous membranes of the rabbit.

In mutagenicity tests in vitro, the chemical does not induce point mutations or chromosome aberrations, nor does it interact with DNA. Further mutagenicity investigations are currently being carried out on behalf of the US Department of Health and Human Services.

## 2. Name of substance

| | | |
|---|---|---|
| 2.1 | Usual name | m-Chlorobenzotrifluoride |
| 2.2 | IUPAC-name | 3-Chlor-α,α,α-trifluortoluene |
| 2.3 | CAS-No. | 98-15-7 |

## 3. Synonyms, common and trade names

3-Chlorobenzotrifluoride
3-Chloro-α,α,α-trifluortoluol
3-Chloro-1-trifluoromethylbenzene

## 4. Structural and molecular formulae

4.1 Structural formula

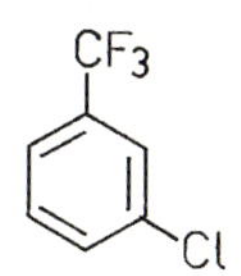


4.2 Molecular formula $C_7H_4ClF_3$

## 5. Physical and chemical properties

| | | |
|---|---|---|
| 5.1 | Molecular mass, g/mol | 180.6 |
| 5.2 | Melting point, °C | –56 (Hoechst, 1986a) |
| 5.3 | Boiling point, °C | 139.4 (Hoechst, 1986a) |
| 5.4 | Vapour pressure, hPa | 6 (at 20 °C) (Hoechst, 1986a) |
| 5.5 | Density, $g/cm^3$ | 1.34 (at 20 °C) (Hoechst, 1986a) |
| 5.6 | Solubility in water | 91 mg/l (Hoechst, 1986a) |
| 5.7 | Solubility in organic solvents | Completely soluble in all of the usual water-free organic solvents (Hoechst, 1986a) |
| 5.8 | Solubility in fat | No information available |
| 5.9 | pH-value | – |
| 5.10 | Conversion factor | 1 ppm $\hat{=}$ 7.4 $mg/m^3$<br>1 $mg/m^3$ $\hat{=}$ 0.14 ppm<br>(at 25 °C and 1013 hPa) |

## 6. Uses

Intermediate for dyestuffs and pesticides (Sax, 1979; Hoechst, 1986a).

## 7. Experimental results

7.1 Toxicokinetics and metabolism
No information available.

7.2 Acute and subacute toxicity

Groups of 5 male and 5 female Wistar rats [HOE:WISKF (SPF71)strain] with average body weights of 194 g and 179 g respectively were given m-chlorobenzotrifluoride by stomach tube at doses of 3150 and 5000 mg/kg body weight. At 3150 mg/kg, no deaths occurred in either the males or the females during the 14-day observation period. After administration of 5000 mg/kg, 1 of the 5 males and 2 of the 5 females died. Symptoms of toxicity in the surviving rats included reduced spontaneous activity, drawn-in flanks, crouching or cringing postures, irregular breathing, ruffled fur, lying on the side or belly, stilted or reeling gait and forward movements. Additional symptoms observed in the 5000 mg/kg group were abnormal breathing sounds, jerky breathing, increased frequency of breathing, uncoordinated gait, obvious eye-watering, partly-closed or closed eyes and discoloration of the edges of the eyelids and the snout. The females were free of symptoms 5 days after treatment, and the males 6 days after treatment. Body weight gain was not impaired. Macroscopic investigation of the animals which died revealed that in one of the females the gut was full of a yellow substance and the liver was a lighter colour. The rats killed at the end of the observation period were without macroscopic findings (Hoechst, 1986c).

## 7.3 Skin and mucous membrane effects

Neat m-chlorobenzotrifluoride (0.5 ml) was applied semiocclusively to the shaved dorsal skin of 3 New Zealand albino rabbits. The application site was evaluated 30 and 60 minutes and 24, 48 and 72 hours after the patch was removed. As some symptoms were still visible after 72 hours, additional evaluations were made after 7 and 14 days. Slight to clear localized erythema was evident in all animals 60 minutes to 7 days after removal of the patch, and very slight oedema was present in 2 animals 72 hours after the chemical was applied. In addition, the skin of all of the rabbits was dry, chapped and scaly 7 days after the application, and 2 rabbits still had dry, chapped skin 14 days after treatment. The erythema and oedema were no longer visible after 14 days. Based on these findings, the substance was classified as non-irritating to rabbit skin (Hoechst, 1986b).

To test the irritancy of m-chlorobenzotrifluoride to the mucous membranes, 3 New Zealand albino rabbits had 0.1 ml of the substance instilled into the conjunctival sac of the left eye. The untreated right eyes served as controls. The treated eyes were rinsed out thoroughly with physiological saline, 24 hours after instillation of the test substance, and at subsequent examination times when the eyes were still producing secretions or when a corneal investigation with fluorescein sodium solution took place. The eyes were examined 1, 24, 48 and 72 hours after instillation of the test substance. At 24 and 72 hours, the cornea was inspected for damage under UV light following instillation of a drop of 0.01% fluorescein sodium solution into the eye. One hour after instillation, corneal swelling was seen, as well as clear hyperaemia of some corneal blood vessels and crimson coloration of the cornea. The cornea of one rabbit was still slightly swollen and crimson-coloured 24 hours after instillation, whilst at 48 hours the same rabbit had only hyperaemia of some of the conjunctival blood vessels. None of the animals showed any irritant effects 72 hours after instillation. Based on these findings, m-chlorobenzotrifluoride was classified as non-irritating to rabbit eyes (Hoechst, 1986a).

7.4 Sensitization

No information available.

7.5 Subchronic and chronic toxicity

No information available.

7.6 Genotoxicity

7.6.1 In vitro

m-Chlorobenzotrifluoride was tested for point-mutagenic effets in the Salmonella/microsome test in strains TA 98, TA 100, TA 1535, TA 1537 and TA 1538. The study was carried out with and without metabolic activation. The concentrations tested were 50, 100 and 500 μg/plate. There was no evidence of point-mutagenic activity in any of the 5 strains, whether S9-mix was added or not (Mazza et al., 1986).

A further Salmonella/microsome test was performed in strains TA 98, TA 100, TA 1535, TA 1537 and TA 1538 as well as in Escherichia coli strain WP2, to determine whether m-chlorobenzotrifluoride was point-mutagenic. The study was carried out with and without metabolic activation. Concentrations of 10, 33.3, 100, 333.3, 1000 and 5000 μg/plate were used. m-Chlorobenzotrifluoride had no point-mutagenic effect in *Salmonella typhimurium* or *Escherichia coli*, either with or without the addition of S9-mix (CCR, 1988a).

This result was stated in a comparable Test (Salmonella (microsometest with preincubation) on Salmonella typhimurium TA 97, TA 98, TA 100, TA 1535 and TA 1537 (Zeiger, 1988).

m-Chlorobenzotrifluoride was tested for its ability to induce chromosomal aberrations in Chinese Hamster V79 cells in vitro. Cultures of V79 cells were treated with the test substance at the following doses for 4 hours: 5, 25, 50 and 150 μg/ml without S9-mix; 20, 400 and 800 μg/ml with S9-mix. Processing of the cultures took place 7, 18 and 28 hours after addition of the test substance. m-Chlorobenzotrifluoride did not induce chromosomal aberrations in V79 cells in vitro (CCR, 1988b).

In Bacillus subtilis (strains PB 1652 and PB 1791) the possible DNA-damaging effect of m-chlorobenzotrifluoride was studied by the soft agar method (standard protocol). Sterile paper discs (9 mm diameter) impregnated with 30 µl of the chemical were placed in the middle of agar plates on which the strains were established. After incubation for 24 hours at 37 °C, the zones of growth inhibition around the discs were measured. m-Chlorobenzotrifluoride did not induce DNA damage (Mazza et al., 1986).

m-Chlorobenzotrifluoride was further tested in *Saccharomyces cerevisiae* (strain 6117) with and without the addition of S9-mix, at a concentration of 2000 µg/ml. There were no signs of crossing-over or gene conversion (Mazza et al., 1986).

7.6.2 In vivo

No information available.

7.7 Carcinogenicity

No information available.

7.8 Reproductive toxicity

No information available.

7.9 Effects on the immune system

No information available.

7.10 Neurotoxicity

No information available.

7.11 Other effects

No information available.

## 8. Experience in humans

No information available.

## 9. Threshold limit values

No information available.

## References

CCR (Cytotest Cell Research GmbH & Co KG)
*Salmonella typhimurium* and *Escherichia coli* reverse mutation assay with m-chlorobenzotrifluoride
Project 115817 (1988a)
Commissioned by BG Chemie

CCR (Cytotest Cell Research GmbH & Co KG
Chromosome aberration assay in Chinese hamster V79 cells in vitro with m-chlorobenzotrifluoride
Project 115828 (1988b)
Commissioned by BG Chemie

Hoechst AG, Pharma Forschung Toxikologie
m-Chlorbenzotrifluorid – Prüfung auf Augenreizung am Kaninchen
Unpublished report no. 86.0543 (1986a)

Hoechst AG, Pharma Forschung Toxikologie
m-Chlorbenzotrifluorid – Prüfung auf Hautreizung am Kaninchen
Unpublished report no. 86.0591 (1986b)

Hoechst AG, Pharma Forschung Toxikologie
m-Chlorbenzotrifluorid – Prüfung der akuten oralen Toxizität an der männlichen und weiblichen Wistar-Ratte
Unpublished report no. 86.0639 (1986c)

Mazza, G., Dacarro, C., Bonferoni, C., Bonferoni, B.
Studies on the mutagenic activity of benzotrifluoride and 12 derivatives in microbial short term assays
Farmaco (prat.), 41, 215–225 (1986)

Sax, I. (ed.)
Dangerous Properties of Industrial Materials
5th ed.
van Nostrand Reinhold Co. (1979)

Zeiger, E.
Salmonella/microsome Test with m-Chlorobenzotrifluoride peronal Communication, March, 22 (1988)
Department of health and human services, Research Triangle Park, N.C. 27709

# Terephthalic acid

## 1. Summary and assessment

Terephthalic acid (TPA) is rapidly excreted via the urine and faeces after single and repeated administration by a number of routes. It does not accumulate in the tissues and there is only slight absorption through the skin and mucous membranes.

TPA is slightly toxic after acute administration $LD_{50}$ rat oral 1960 mg/kg or >5000 mg/kg; mouse 1470 or >5000 mg/kg). It is not irritating to the skin or mucous membranes.

Repeated administration of high doses of TPA (from 3.7 g/kg/day) to young rats results in increased calcium secretion and bladder stone formation. Hyperplasia of the bladder wall epithelium occurs as a consequence of irritation by the bladder stones, but there are no indications of neoplasia. In rats and guinea-pigs, inhalation of 10 mg TPA/$m^3$ air, as a dust, for 6 months has not resulted in any toxicologically significant effects.

The formation of bladder stones, and the effects on the bladder epithelium (hyperplasia, papilloma, metaplasia and, to a small extent, carcinoma development) are generally not observed until the last quarter of the long-term studies, and are attributed mainly to the irritant action of the bladder stones (Heck and Tyl, 1985).

TPA is not mutagenic in the Salmonella/microsome test.

In the rat, TPA is embryotoxic, causing foetal death and reduced vitality or survival rate.

In man, no cases of poisoning, damage to the organs or skin irritation are known so far as a result of prolonged handling of the substance.

## 2. Name of substance

| | | |
|---|---|---|
| 2.1 | Usual name | Terephthalic acid |
| 2.2 | IUPAC-name | 1,4-benzene dicarbonic acid |
| 2.3 | CAS-No. | 100-21-0 |

## 3. Synonyms, common and trade names

Benzene-1,4-dicarbonic acid
1,4-Benzene dicarboxylic acid
p-Benzene dicarboxylic acid
TPS
TPA
Terephthalsäure

## 4. Structural and molecular formulae

4.1 Structural formula

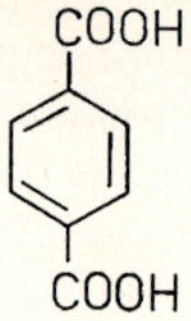


4.2 Molecular formula $C_8H_6O_4$

## 5. Physical and chemical properties

| | | |
|---|---|---|
| 5.1 | Molecular mass g/mol | 166.13 |
| 5.2 | Melting point, °C | Sublimates (300 °C) (Hoffmann and Mayer, 1982) |
| 5.3 | Boiling point, °C | >300 (Sublimation) (Hoffmann and Mayer, 1982) |
| 5.4 | Vapour pressure, hPa | <0.01 (at 20 °C) (Hoffmann and Mayer, 1982)<br>5.3 (at 150 °C)<br>20 (at 200 °C)<br>200 (at 250 °C)<br>930 (at 300 °C)<br>(Hoffmann and Mayer, 1982) |
| 5.5 | Density, $g/cm^3$ | 1.51 (at 20 °C) (Hoffmann and Mayer, 1982) |
| 5.6 | Solubility in water | 0.0019 g/100 g (at 25 °C) (Hoffmann and Mayer, 1982) |
| 5.7 | Solubility in organic solvents | Dimethyl acetamide (>10% at 25 °C)<br>Tetramethyl urea (>10% at 25 °C) |

| | |
|---|---|
| | Dimethyl formamide (7.5% at 25 °C)<br>Pyridine<br>Dimethyl sulphoxide<br>Methanol (0.2% at 25 °C)<br>(Hoffmann and Mayer, 1982) |
| 5.8 Solubility in fat | No information available |
| 5.9 pH-value | No information available |
| 5.10 Conversion factor | 1 ppm $\hat{=}$ 6.79 mg/m$^3$<br>1 mg/m$^3$ $\hat{=}$ 0.15 ppm<br>(at 25 °C and 1013 hPa) |
| 5.11 Distribution coefficient (log P, 1-octanol/water) | 1.96<br>(Dunn and Johansson, 1983) |

## 6. Uses

Starting material for manufacturing polyesters (Hoffmann and Mayer, 1982)

## 7. Experimental results

7.1 Toxicokinetics and metabolism

A study of the absorption, distribution and excretion of $^{14}$C-TPA after oral, intratracheal and dermal exposure in male rats, and after ocular application in male rabbits produced the following results (Moffit et al., 1975): After oral administration of a single dose (40 and 80 mg TPA/animal), over 80% of the radioactivity administered was excreted within 48 hours, of which approx. 40% was in the urine, and approx. 47% in the faeces. A similar excretion pattern was found after repeated administration of the same doses of TPA (five times within 10 days). Over 90% of the administered dose was present in the urine und faeces, with less than 0.1% in the liver, lungs, heart, kidneys, spleen, adrenal glands, pancreas, testes, brain and femur. After intratracheal administration of 5 and 10 mg $^{14}$C-TPA/animal, 45.7 to 66.6% of the radioactivity was found in the urine after 48 hours, and only small quantities (3.4 to 6.4%) in the faeces. $^{14}$C-Activities of the same order were found in the urine and faces after repeated intratracheal administration of the same doses (five times within 10 days). Less than 1% was measurable in the lungs and the tracheal lymph nodes, and less than 0.1% in the other organs examined (liver, heart, kidneys, spleen, adrenal glands, pancreas, testes, brain and femur). After covered dermal application of $^{14}$C-TPA to the shaved dorsal skin of rats (80 mg in 0.2 ml of aqueous Triton X-solution, applied once or five times within 10 days), 5.1% of the applied activity was found after single administration for 24 hours and subsequent washing, with 1.6% being present in the urine, 0.6% in the faeces, 1.9% on the treated skin, 0.7% in the liver and 0.3% in all the other organs assessed (lungs, heart, kidneys, spleen, adrenal glands, pancreas, testes, brain, femur). After repeated covered application over 10 days, 9.4% of the administered activity was measured 24 hours after the last application (4.3% in the urine, 2.2% in the faeces and 2.1% in the other organs). TPA was not irritating to the skin. A dose of 50 mg $^{14}$C-TPA was instilled into the conjunctival sacs of rabbits' eyes,and washed out with distilled water after 5 minutes in one test group and after 24 hours in a second group. After 5 minutes of contact, 1.8% was excreted in the urine within 10 days, 0.5% in the faeces, and less than 0.1% in the eye and all other organs (same organs as for the other application methods). Even after 24 hours of contact, only small quantities of TPA were absorbed. Within 10 days 6.1% of the applied activity was detectable in the urine, 2.2% in the faeces and less than 0.1% in the other organs, including the eye. After urinary extraction with a chloroform-methanol mixture, the $^{14}$C activity was found mainly in the aqueous fraction (Moffit et al., 1975).

After thin-layer chromatographic tests by Hoshi and Kuretani (1967), orally-administered $^{14}$C-TPA (85 mg/kg, specific activity 2 μCi/mg, Wistar King A rats) was not metabolised and was excreted unchanged in the urine: within 48 hours, 93.8% of the dose was detectable in the urine and 3.3% in the faeces. There is a discrepancy here with the results of the studies carried out by Moffit et al. (1975).

In further studies on toxicokinetics and metabolism, young F-344 rats (males, 200 to 350 g, females 140 to 225 g) were given $^{14}$C-labelled TPA (25 μCi), intravenously or orally (by stomach tube). The urinary excretion of TPA and its metabolites was determined, as was the half-life of the labelled TPA in the plasma. After intravenous injection, the plasma half-life was 1.2 hours (±0.4 hours), whilst after oral administration the half-life was slightly longer (2.43 hours). The kinetic study showed that after intravenous injection almost 100% of the TPA was excreted unchanged in the urine within 8 hours, with no metabolism of the substance. The rate of elimination after oral administration has not been reported (Wolkowski-Tyl et al., 1982).

Laying hens (17- to 18-months-old, weight 2 to 4 kg, ABRA strain) were infused continuously with $^{14}C$-labelled TPA, via the renal portal circulation. Between five and eight urine samples were taken at 10-minute intervals from each kidney, approx. 50 minutes from the start of infusion. Over 85% of the $^{14}C$-labelled TPA was found in the urine. The majority (60%) was excreted in the „first pass" directly via the kidney (Tremaine and Quebbemann, 1985).

## 7.2 Acute and subacute toxicity

In the male rat (strain not indicated) the oral $LD_{50}$ exceeded 5000 mg/kg. None of the nine animals given 5000 mg/kg died within a 28-day observation period. On intraperitoneal injection the $LD_{50}$ was 2250 mg/kg (no further details; Massmann, 1966).

A group of 10–20 female Wistar rats (weight 210±10 g) were given TPA by stomach tube, and the resultant $LD_{50}$ was 1960 mg/kg body weight. After intraperitoneal injection to a comparable group of animals, an $LD_{50}$ of 1210 mg/kg body weight was obtained, and after intravenous injection a dose of 1000 mg/kg body weight was not found to be lethal (Caujolle et al., 1966).

The acute oral $LD_{50}$ of TPA in the mouse was >5000 mg/kg after a 3-day observation period; on intraperitoneal injection it was 1430 (1240–1650) mg/kg (Hoshi et al., 1968).

Five male Swiss mice (weight approx. 20 g) each received an intraperitoneal injection of TPA in 0.5% methyl cellulose, at dose levels of 200, 400, 800, 1200, 1600, 2400 and 3200 mg/kg body weight. The $LD_{50}$ determined from this was 1900 (1583–2280) mg/kg body weight (Grigas et al., 1971).

Female Swiss mice (weight 24±2 g) were given TPA by stomach tube, and an $LD_{50}$ of 1470 mg/kg body weight was determined. Intraperitoneal and intravenous administration to comparable animals resulted in $LD_{50}$ values of 880 and 770 mg/kg body weight, respectively. Over-excitement and increased aggression were observed in the rats and mice which died during the study, whilst animals which received sublethal doses showed practically no symptoms (Caujolle et al., 1966).

The intravenous administration of TPA (2 mg/kg/min.) to seven mongrels resulted in a lethal dose of 767 mg/kg body weight (Grigas et al., 1971).

The oral administration of high doses of TPA in the feed (at concentrations of 0.5, 1.5, 3.0, 4.0 and 5.0%) to young, weaned male and female rats (Fischer-344, 28 days old) for 2 weeks resulted in weight loss, at the two highest doses and, at a dietary level of 3 to 5% (3.7 to 5.7 g/kg/day), a dose-related increase in bladder stone formation. At the highest TPA concentration, roughly 95% of all the males and 75% of all the females had one or more bladder stones. Hyperplasia of the bladder wall epithelium and haematuria occurred at the same time, but histological changes in the bladder were found only in animals with bladder stones (Chin et al., 1981).

Young male Fischer-344 rats (age 28 days) received 4% TPA per day in their feed for 2 weeks. They showed a 20% reduction in body weight compared with the controls. At autopsy, bladder stones were found in 50% of the animals, most of these stones being located in the lumen of the bladder, with some in the ureter or in the renal pelvis. There was marked hyperacidity of the urine. Blood tests revealed increased calcium and magnesium levels, and the excretion of these elements in the urine had also increased (Wolkowski-Tyl and Chin, 1983).

Repeated inhalation of 25 mg TPA/m$^3$ air for 6 hours per day, 5 day/week for 4 weeks caused no toxicologically significant effects in rats (no further data; Bemis et al., 1982).

Ten male and ten female rats (strain not indicated) were exposed to TPA dust for 6 hours/day, 5 days/week for 4 weeks at concentrations of 0, 0.52, 1.19 and 3.31 mg/m$^3$ air. Lung function tests were carried out on six rats/sex in the highest exposure group and in the control group. There were no deaths and no symptoms of toxicity during the study, and macroscopic investigation did not reveal any effects. Body weights, haematological and clinical-chemical tests demonstrated no significant differences between the treated and untreated animals. Histopathological examination revealed degeneration of the tracheal epithelium in 19/20 rats in the highest exposure group, compared with 1/20 in the control group. However, under normal and difficult breathing conditions the lung function tests (pulmonary ventilation, transpulmonary pressure, residual volume, compliance, resistance, respiration rate and minute volume) showed no differences between the groups. The highest concentration of 3.31 mg/m$^3$ air per day was considered by the authors to be the no-effect-level (Jernigan et al., 1988).

7.3 Skin and mucous membrane effects

As part of the aforementioned metabolism study on rats, it was shown that TPA did not cause skin irritation after single (24-hour) or multiple (10-day) applications (Moffit et al., 1975).

A 15% TPA suspension in olive oil was tolerated in rabbits' eyes without irritation (no further data; Massmann, 1966). The TPA concentration was too low for this result to be of much value.

7.4 Sensitization

According to screening tests in the Industrial Medicine Laboratory of Eastman Kodak, TPA is not a sensitizer (no further data, cited in Moffit et al., 1975).

7.5 Subchronic and chronic toxicity

Ten female rats (strain not indicated) received an intraperitoneal injection of a 15% TPA suspension in olive oil (0.3 to 0.6 ml/animal) every 7 days for 102 days. The total dose was 1.1 g/animal. During this time none of the animals showed any marked changes in appearance. After the test all the animals were dissected, but there were no pathological findings. Compared with the control animals, the weight development of the treated animals was retarded from the 6th week onwards (Massmann, 1966).

Weaned male and female rats, 28 days old (origin Wistar, body weight 56 and 55 g, respectively), received TPA in their feed for 13 weeks, at a concentration of 5% in the first week and 3% for the remaining 12 weeks. Dissection of the treated animals revealed bladder stones in 11/18 males and 3/19 females after 90 days. Slight to moderate hyperplasia of the bladder epithelium was found in 13/18 males and 3/19 females. There were no indications of neoplastic changes. There was a close correlation between the occurrence of bladder stones and the development of bladder hyperplasia: 62% of the males (8/13) and 100% of the females (3/3) displaying transitional epithelial hyperplasia also had bladder stones (Vogin, 1972).

In a further 90-day feeding study, male and female Wistar and Sprague Dawley rats received 0.03, 0.125, 0.5, 2.0 and 5.0% TPA in their feed. The rats were 15 to 17 weeks old. The median body weight of Wistar rats was 400 g for the males and 620 g for the females, that of the Sprague-Dawley rats was 420 g for the males and 305 g for the females. The male Wistar rats in this age group were much more sensitive than the male Sprague-Dawley rats in terms of bladder stone formation. In the Wistar rats, bladder stones occurred in 1/5 males in the 5% dose group after 30 days, in 1/10 males in the 0.03% dose group after 90 days, and in 4/10 males in the 5% group after 90 days. Throughout the exposure period none of the male Sprague-Dawley rats developed bladder stones. The stones were also observed in 1/10 female Wistar rats, and in 1/10 female Sprague-Dawley rats in the highest dose group after 90 days. The findings on the bladder (slight to moderate hyperplasia of the transitional epithelium) also ocurred in this test arrangement, with hyperplasia being observed after 90 days in 3/9 male and 5/10 female Wistar rats, and in 1/10 male and 4/10 female Sprague-Dawley rats. The correlation between bladder stone formation and hyperplasia was not as distinct as in the study described above (Ledoux et al., 1982).

In a subchronic inhalation study, male Sprague-Dawley rats and male Hartley guinea-pigs were exposed to a TPA dust at a concentration of 10 $mg/m^3$ air for 5 days/week, 6 hours per day, for a period of 6 months. The test parameters (body weight, organ weights, clinical chemistry or urine analyses, macroscopic and histopathological examination of the tissues), indicated no toxicologically significant modifications (Lewis et al., 1982).

## 7.6 Genotoxicity

As part of a study on the mutagenic potential of tobacco smoke, TPA ws tested on four strains of *Salmonella typhimirium* (TA 98, TA 100, TA 1535 and TA 1537), with and without metabolic activation, at doses of up to 3 μmol/plate. Under these test conditions TPA showed no point-mutagenic activity (Florin et al., 1980).

In a further study, TPA was tested on *Salmonella typhimurium* strains TA 98, TA 100, TA 1535 and TA 1537, with and without a metabolising system (from Aroclor-induced rat or hamster livers), at dose levels of 0.1 to 10 mg/plate. Again, under these test conditions, TPA was not shown to be point-mutagenic (Zeiger et al., 1982).

## 7.7 Carcinogenicity

In an inadequately-documented study, rats received up to 5% TPA in their feed for 2 years. There were no indications of carcinogenicity (Du Pont, 1975).

Male and female Wistar rats (initial weight and age of the animals were not indicated) received TPA in their feed at concentrations of 1, 2 or 5%, for 2 years. Bladder stones were found during the study in 42/47 males and 39/42 females in the high-dose group, and in 1/48 females in the low-dose group. No bladder stones were found in males or females in the median-dose group, in males in the low-dose group or in the control animals. Bladder and ureter neoplasms occurred in 21/37 males and 21/34 females in the high-dose group, in 1/48 males and 2/47 females in the median-dose group, and in 1/43 males in the low-dose group. No urogenital neoplasms were found in the low-dose females or in the controls. The author concludes that the presence of the stones leads to changes in the epithelium of the urinary tract, with increased incidences of hyperplasia, papillomas, squamous metaplasia, transitional cell tumours and squamous cell carcinomas (Gross, 1974).

In a further 2-year feeding study, male and female F-344 rats received 20, 142 or 1000 mg TPA/kg daily for 2 years. The initial age of the animals was 7 weeks, the body weight of the males being 135 to 179 g and that of the females being 199 to 224 g. Intermediate dissection after 6 and 12 months revealed no stones in the urogenital tract. After 18 months 2/27 females in the high-dose group, but none of the males, had developed gritty particles or bladder stones. During the last 6 months and at the end of the study, bladder stones were found only in the high-dose females (11/86), the relatively low incidence of bladder stones being attributed to the fact that the TPA dose was low. The histopathological examination of the bladders was carried out by two different teams. Whilst one team found transitional cell adenomas of the bladder after 18 months in 2/27 females in the high-dose group, one of these findings was diagnosed by the other institute as epithelial hyperplasia. At the end of the study, one team found transitional cell adenomas in 15/79 females in the high-dose group whilst the other team found them in 10/73 high-dose females. One female in the control group also displayed this finding. No transitional epithelial adenomas were found in any of the treated males. Four of the transitional cell adenomas diagnosed in the high-dose females were diagnosed as hyperplasia by the other team. A further lesion was described as an adenoma by one team and as a metastasising carcinoma by the other. Transitional cell carcinomas were only diagnosed in females of the high-dose group (2/79 and 1/73). Hyperplasia of the mucous membrane of the bladder was found in the high-dose females (14/79 and 23/73), but only in a very small number of high-dose males, if any (2/82 and 0/80). This effect was also observed in females and males in the median-dose group (2/70 and 3/82, respectively), and in females and males in the low-dose group (7/76 and 9/82), respectively). However, 8/83 female controls and 2/87 male controls also displayed this finding (CIIT, 1983).

7.8 Reproductive toxicity

Ledoux et al. (1982) gave female and male Wistar and CD rats concentrations of 0.03, 0.125, 0.5, 2 and 5% of TPA in their feed for 90 days. Ten pairs per concentration group were then formed, and these continued to receive the corresponding TPA concentration in the feed during the periods of mating, pregnancy, lactation and rearing. Although the fertility index and the litter size in the Wistar rats were higher than in the CD rats, TPA did not appear to exert any influence on these end-points, and the authors concluded that reproduction had not been affected in the parent animals. By contrast, the foetuses and newborn animals in the 2 and 5% dose groups displayed marked effects. In these two concentration groups, 76% of the Wistar rats and 96% of the CD rats were still-born. The post-natal lethality in Wistar and CD rats was 50%. The body weights of the newborn Wistar rats in the highest dose group were significantly lower than those of the control group on day 1 and 21, whilst the same was true for the newborn CD rats on day 21 (Ledoux et al., 1982).

After administration of TPA in the feed of male chickens at concentrations of 0.1 to 0.4%, other investigators found atrophy of the interstitial cells of the testes. Syncytial giant cells and secondary spermatocytal giant cells were found in many parts of the seminiferous tubules, and delayed spermatogenesis was also observed (no further data; Kono and Nakajima, 1965).

7.9 Effects on the immune system

No information available.

7.10 Neurotoxicity

No information available.

7.11 Other effects

Two further authors observed that after inhalation exposure of rats to TPA, the uptake of noradrenaline and choline in the synapses of the cerebral cortices of rats was inhibited (extract from Russian abstract, no further data, Shevchenko, 1982; Davidenko, 1984).

After administering a 0.5% TPA diet for 7 days to Swiss albino mice (815 mg/kg/day), no changes were observed, kidney function was normal (phenol red test, measurement in the plasma). After a single intraperitoneal injection of 25, 50, 100 or 200 mg TPA/kg, phenol red excretion by the renal tubules was unaffected. At dose levels of 300, 500 and 1000 mg/kg, however, the phenol red concentration in the plasma had increased significantly (58.2, 65.6 and

85.6 μg/ml plasma, respectively, as opposed to 31.4 μg/ml plasma in the control animals; Hoshi et al., 1968).

The SGOT and SGPT activities in the plasma of mice which had received 801 mg TPA/kg/day (0.5% TPA) in their feed for 7 days, were not modified (Hoshi et al., 1968).

In mice given 852 mg TPA/kg/day (0.5% TPA) in their feed for 7 days, a subsequent bromosulphthalein test revealed a significantly lower bromosulphthalein concentration in the treated animals compared with the controls (6.3 mg/ml as opposed to 10.4 mg/ml). TPA therefore appears to accelerate bromosulphthalein excretion (Hoshi et al., 1968).

After a 0.5% TPA diet was administered to Wistar-King-A rats for 7 days (310 mg/kg/day), the determination of blood sugar, protein, amino acid nitrogen and urea nitrogen revealed no changes relative to controls (Hoshi et al., 1968).

In Swiss albino mice (20 animals treated, 35 controls) the barbiturate sleeping time (40 mg pentobarbital/kg) was reduced from $10.2 \pm 4.0$ minutes in the controls to $6.6 \pm 2.4$ minutes in the treated animals given a 0.5% TPA diet for 7 days (766 mg/kg/day). This reduction was due to enzyme induction in the liver by TPA (Hoshi et al., 1968).

A 4% TPA diet given to rats for 2 weeks led to a reduction in the pH value of the urine, from 6.3 to 5.7 in the males and from 6.2 to 5.7 in the females, as well as to an increase in the calcium excretion from 5.5 mM to 22.2 mM in the males and from 4.9 mM to 23.5 mM in the females. On this 4% TPA diet, 81 mM TPA was measured in the urine of the males and 101 mM in that of females (Chin et al., 1981).

## 8. Experience in humans

An oily paste of TPA (80%) had no irritating action when applied 10 times to the same area of skin. Moreover, this paste was tolerated after 24 hours continuous action without any indications of irritation or reddening (no further data; Massmann, 1966).

## 9. Threshold values

No information available.

## References

Bemis, A.G., Dindorf, J.A., Horwood, B., Samans, C.
Phthalic acid and other benzenepolycarboxylic acids
In: Kirk-Othmer, Encyclopedia of Chemical Technology, 17, 732–777 (1982)

Caujolle, F., Caujolle, D., Moisand, C.
Toxicités comparés des acides nitrobenzoiques pour la souris et le rat
Comptes Rendus, 160, 1097–1100 (1966)

CIIT (Chemical Industry Institute of Toxicology)
Chronic dietary administration of terephthalic acid
Life Science Research Division, CIIT Docket 20124 (1983)

Chin, T.Y., Tyl, R.W., Popp, J.A., Heck, H. d'A.
Chemical urolithiasis
Toxicol. Appl. Pharmacol., 58, 307–321 (1981)

Du Pont de Nemours Co., Haskell Laboratories
Data Sheet 9/25/75, Wilmington (1975)
cited in: Hoffmann and Mayer (1982)

Davidenko, A.V., Vasilev, A.N., Kucherenko, N.E.
Inhibition of active capture of $^{14}C$ noradrenaline and $^{3}H$-choline in cortex synaptosomes in rats after inhalation exposure to TPA
Ukr. Biokhim. Zh., 54, 211–213 (1982)

Davidenko, A.V.
Chronic effects of terephthalic acid on synaptosomes in rat brain
Biol. Nauki, 1, 31–34 (1984)

Dunn, W.J., Johansson, E.
Nonadditivity of 1-octanol/water partition coefficients of disubstituted benzenes
Quant. Struct.-Act. Relat., 2, 156–163 (1983)

Florin, J., Rutberg, L., Curvall, M., Enzell, C.R.
Screening of tobacco smoke constituents for mutagenicity using the Ames-Test
Toxicology, 18, 219–232 (1980)

Grigas, E.O., Ruiz, R., Aviado, D.M.
Cardiopulmonary effects of antimalarial drugs
Toxicol. Appl. Pharmacol., 18, 469–486 (1971)

Gross, J.
The effects of prolonged feeding of terephthalic acid (TPA) to rats
Agricultural Research Service (1974)
reviewed in Chin et al., (1981)

Heck, H. d'A., Tyl, R.W.
The induction of bladder stones by terephthalic acid, dimethylterephthalate and melamine (2,4,6-triamino-s-triazine) and its relevance to risk assessment
Regul. Toxicol. Pharmacol., 5, 294–313 (1985)

Hodgman, C.E. (ed.)
Handbook of Chemistry and Physics
30th ed., pp. 1054–1055
Chemical Rubber Publishing Co., Cleveland OH. (1947)

Hoshi, A., Kuretani, K.
Metabolism of terephthalic acid
Chem. Pharm. Bull., 15, 1979–1984 (1967)

Hoshi, A., Yanai, R., Kuretani, K.
Toxicity of terephthalic acid
Chem. Pharm. Bull., 16, 1655–1660 (1968)

Jernigan, J.D., Leach, C.L., Hatoum, N.S., Talsma, D.M., Garvin, P.J.
Four week inhalation study of terephthalic acid
The Toxicologist, 8, 252 (1988)

Kono, K., Nakajima, E.
Effect of terephthalic acid on the viscera of chickens
Nippon Kakin Gakkaishi, 2, 205–219 (1965)
reviewed in Chem. Abstr. 66:44562b

Ledoux, T.A., Reel, J.R., Gralla, E.J.
A ninety-day study of terephthalic acid-induced urolithiasis and reproductive performance in Wistar and CD rats, final report, FYI-OTS-0482-0190
Environmental Protection Agency, US (1982)

Lewis, T.R., Lynch, D.W., Schuler, R.L.
Absence of urinary bladder and kidney toxicity in rats and guinea pigs exposed to inhaled terephthalic acid and dimethyl terephthalate
The Toxicologist, 2, 7 (1982)

Massmann, W.
Gewerbehygienisch-toxikologisches Gutachen über p-Toluylsäuremethylester, Dimethylterephthalat und Terephthalsäure
Institut für Arbeitsmedizin der Universität Tübingen, 26. 2. 1966

Moffit, A.E., Clary, J.J., Lewis, T.R., Blanck, M.D., Perone, V.B.
Absorption, distribution and excretion of terephthalic acid and dimethylterephthalate
Am. Ind. Hyg. Assoc. J., 36, 633–641 (1975)

Tremaine, L.M., Quebbemann, A.J.
The renal handling of terephthalic acid
Toxicol. Appl. Pharmacol., 77, 165–174 (1985)

Hoffmann, G., Mayer, D.
Terephthalsäure mit Isophthalsäure
in Ullmanns Enzyklopädie der technischen Chemie
4th ed., Volume 22, p. 519–528
Verlag Chemie, Weinheim (1982)

Vogin, E.E. (1972)
Subacute feeding studies (13 week) in rats with dimethyl terephthalate, isophthalic acid and terephthalic acid
reviewed by Heck, H.d'A., Tyl, R.W. (1985)

Wolkowski-Tyl, R., Chin, T.Y.
Effects of selected therapeutic agents on urolithiasis induced by terephthalic acid in the male weanling Fischer 344 rat
Fundam. Appl. Toxicol., 3, 552–558 (1983)

Wolkowski-Tyl, R., Chin, T.Y., Heck, H. d'A.
Chemical urolithiasis (part III)
Drug Metab. Dispos., 10, 486–490 (1982)

Zeiger, E., Haworth, S., Speck, W., Mortelmans, K.
Phthalate ester testing in the National Toxicology Program's environmental mutagenesis test development program
Environ. Health Perspect., 45, 99–101 (1982)

# Isopropyl ethylene glycol ether

## 1. Summary and assessment

In rats and dogs, isopropyl ethylene glycol ether and its metabolites are essentially eliminated in the urine (more than 70%) and to a slight extent in the exhaled breath (ca. 14%). Isopropoxyacetic acid and its glycine conjugate are obtained as metabolites.

The acute toxicity of the substance is slight when administered orally, dermally or by inhalation (rats, oral $LD_{50}$ 5.66 ml/kg; rats, inhalation $LC_{50}$ 8,200 mg/m$^3$; mouse, oral $LD_{50}$ 2,300 mg/kg; rabbit, dermal $LD_{50}$ 1.6 ml/kg). In animal tests, particularly after inhalation exposure, there is increased decomposition of erythrocytes, a reduction in haemoglobin, compensatory reticulocytosis, and haemoglobinuria and haematuria. In addition, after acute inhalation exposure there are indications of kidney impairment, whilst after sub-acute inhalation exposure at concentrations ranging from 100 to 1,000 ppm, the spleen is the target organ, correlating with the haematological findings. After repeated inhalation exposure at low concentrations (10 or 30 ppm), no damage has been observed.

Isopropyl ethylene glycol ether has a slight irritating effect on the skin of animals but a clear irritating effect on their eyes, and may bring about corneal opacities.

Teratogenic action has been detected with other monoalkyl ethylene glycol ethers in tests on rats and rabbits, but this is not the case for isopropyl ethylene glycolether, which has shown evidence of a slight foetotoxic effect in both species, particularly at maternally-toxic doses.

## 2. Name of substance

| | | |
|---|---|---|
| 2.1 | Usual name | Isopropyl ethylene glycol ether |
| 2.2 | IUPAC-name | 4-Methyl-3-oxapentan-1-ol |
| 2.3 | CAS-No. | 109-59-1 |

## 3. Synonyms, common and trade names

Isopropylethylenglykolether
Ethylene glycol isopropyl ether
Ethylene glycol monoisopropyl ether
β-Hydroxyethyl isopropyl ether
2-(1-Methylethoxy)-ethanol
IPEGE
2-Isopropoxyethanol
Isopropyl Cellosolve
Isopropyl glycol
Oxitol

## 4. Structural and molecular formulae

| | | |
|---|---|---|
| 4.1 | Structural formula | $(CH_3)_2CH-O-CH_2-CH_2-OH$ |
| 4.2 | Molecular formula | $C_5H_{12}O_2$ |

## 5. Physical and chemical properties

| | | |
|---|---|---|
| 5.1 | Molecular mass, g/mol | 104.15 |
| 5.2 | Melting point, °C | No information available |
| 5.3 | Boiling point, °C | 144 (Clayton and Clayton, 1982) |
| 5.4 | Vapour pressure, hPa | 6.9 (at 25 °C) (Clayton and Clayton, 1982) |
| 5.5 | Density, $g/cm^3$ | 0.903 (at 20 °C) (Clayton and Clayton, 1982) |
| 5.6 | Solubility in water | Good (Clayton and Clayton, 1982) |
| 5.7 | Solubility in organic solvents | Good in alcohol, ether and acetone (Weast, 1981/1982) |
| 5.8 | Solubility in fat | No information available |
| 5.9 | pH-value | No information available |
| 5.10 | Conversion factor | 1 ppm $\hat{=}$ 4.25 $mg/m^3$<br>1 $mg/m^3$ $\hat{=}$ 0.24 ppm<br>(at 25 °C and 1013 hPa) |

## 6. Uses

Solvent for insecticides, herbicides, colours, oil, fats and waxes (Hutson and Pickering, 1971).

## 7. Experimental results

### 7.1 Toxicokinetics and metabolism

The metabolism of isopropyl ethylene glycol ether (IPEGE) was investigated by $^{14}C$-labelling in the rat and the dog. Groups of six male and six female rats (strain Carworth Farm E; weight 200–250 g) received an intraperitoneal injection of 0.993 mg $^{14}C^1$,$^{14}C^2$-labelled IPEGE (9.55 µCi), in 0.5 ml physiological saline. The rats were kept in metabolic chambers for 4 days. Urine and faeces were collected daily. Expired air was absorbed by means of NaOH. After appropriate treatment, the radioactivity of individual samples was measured by liquid scintillation: 73% of the administered radioactivity was excreted in the urine (71% within the first 24 hours), and 14% was eliminated as carbon dioxide in exhaled air (9% in the first 24 hours). About 10% of the administered radioactivity was still detectable in the rats after 4 days. Isopropoxyacetic acid and its glycine conjugate were detected as metabolites in the urine (30 and 40%, respectively, of the activity in the urine). An adult beagle dog (weight 10 kg) received 715 mg $^{14}C^1$,$^{14}C^2$-labelled IPEGE (14.2 µCi) in physiological saline by intraperitoneal injection. It was then kept for 2 days in a metabolic chamber and the urine was collected. Metabolism in the dog was shown to be comparable to that in the rat. Similarly, the two main metabolites, isopropoxyacetic acid and its glycine conjugate, were detected (Hutson and Pickering, 1971).

### 7.2 Acute and subacute toxicity

The oral $LD_{50}$ value for IPEGE in male rats (Carworth-Wistar) was reported to be 5.66 ml/kg (4.11–7.79 ml/kg ± 1.96 standard deviation) after a 14-day observation period (Smyth et al., 1969).

Mice (strain, age and number not given) received IPEGE in oil. An $LD_{50}$ value of 2300 mg/kg body weight was reported (no further details, Saparmamedov, 1974).

In an inhalation study, mice (white Swiss mice, 16 animals/group) were exposed for 7 hours to various concentrations of IPEGE vapour (high degree of purity), and were observed for up to 3 weeks. The $LC_{50}$ value for IPEGE was calculated as 1930 ppm (8200 mg/m$^3$) after the 3-week observation period. Dyspnoea was the most frequent and marked symptom seen, but other symptoms included inability to move (seen prior to death in mice given a lethal dose level) and analgesia (seen in a few animals). At sublethal doses, haemoglobinuria regularly occurred and isolated cases of clouding of the cornea or lens were observed (detailed information on this was not given). Pathological examination of some of the organs gave the following results: numerous hyaline casts, haemosiderin casts and interstitial nephritis were found in the kidneys of most animals, congestion was seen in the cavernous vessels of the spleen; no effects on the heart, liver or lungs were detected. No quantitative data were given and the concentrations at which particular effects occurred were not specified (Werner et al., 1943a).

Four out of six Carworth-Wistar rats died during the 14-day observation period after a 4-hour inhalation exposure to 4000 ppm (18,600 mg/m$^3$) (no further details; Smyth et al., 1969).

A further unpublished investigation of the acute inhalation toxicity of IPEGE in rats (performed by the Dow Chemical W.) was cited by Clayton and Clayton (1982). The results are summarised in Table 1.

The dermal $LD_{50}$ value for IPEGE in rabbits (no details on strain or number of animals) is 1.6 ml/kg (no further information; Smyth et al., 1969).

The effects of repeated inhalation exposure to IPEGE were studied in rats. A group of 23 Wistar rats inhaled 390 ppm (1800 mg/m$^3$) IPEGE for 7 hours/day for 5 weeks. A control group of 23 rats was maintained under the same housing conditions. Pairs of rats were examined for pathological effects after 1, 3 and 5 weeks of exposure and 1 week after the end of the study. Fifteen animals were examined for effects on weight gain and haematological parameters (erythrocytes, leukocytes, differential blood cell count, reticulocytes and haemoglobin) prior to, during (weeks 1 and 5) and 3 weeks after exposure. Anatomical-pathological and histopathological examinations of the liver, kidneys, heart, spleen, lungs and bones were carried out on these rats 3 weeks after the end of exposure. The behaviour and appearance of all of the animals was normal during the study. Weight gain in the control and treated animals was the same. The following haematological effects were found: up to 1 week after the beginning of exposure, there was a decrease in the number of erythrocytes (from $7.5 \times 10^6/mm^3$ to $6 \times 10^6/mm^3$) and in the haemoglobin level [from 13.3 g/100 ml (8.25 mmol/l) to 10 g/100 ml (6.2 mmol/l)]. Despite further exposure, the values returned to normal at the end of the exposure period. The number of reticulocytes also increased in the first week from 5% to 25%, but again returned to the initial value at the end of exposure, despite continued exposure. Apart from a slight increase in immature granulocytes from 0.5 to 2%, there were no effects on the leukocytes. No visible macroscopic

**Table 1.** Acute inhalation toxicity of IPEGE

| Concentration | Duration of exposure (hours) | Number of dead/exposed animals | Observations |
|---|---|---|---|
| Atmosphere saturated with IPEGE at 100 °C and cooled to room temperature | 7 | 4/4 | Blood in the urine after 3 hours, 1 animal had black, enlarged kidneys at autopsy |
| As above | 4 | 2/3 | Bloody urine immediately after exposure, necrotic and dark-coloured kidneys 3 days after exposure |
| As above | 1 | 0/3 | Bloody urine, kidney damage |
| As above | 0.5 | 0/3 | Bloody urine, questionable kidney damage |
| 160 ppm | 4, 6, 7 | 0/5 | Bloody urine during exposure; autopsy 15 days after exposure: moderate kidney damage |
| 80 ppm | 7 | 0/5 | Slight weight loss, bloody urine; 1 rat dissected immediately after exposure: severe kidney damage, pale-coloured liver, bloody urine in the bladder; 1 rat dissected after 9 days; no visible macroscopic kidney damage |
| 80 ppm | 4 | 0/5 | Questionable evidence of blood in the urine, slight weight loss; 1 rat dissected immediately after exposure: severe kidney damage; 1 rat dissected 1 day after exposures: light kidney damage; 1 rat dissected after 9 days; slight kidney damage |

changes were found at autopsy. On histological examination, haemosiderin deposition was found in the spleen and was still present 3 weeks after exposure had ceased. The treated animals showed a decrease in cytoplasmic density in the livers, the pathological significance of which is unclear.This was no longer detectable 3 weeks after the end of the study. After exposure, an increase in bone marrow fat cells was found in a few animals (number not given), but not in the control animals (Werner et al., 1943b).

In a further study involving inhalation exposure (Gage, 1970), the subacute toxicity of IPEGE (100, 300 and 1000 ppm) was investigated in groups of four male and four female rats (Alderly Park, SPF, body weight ca. 200 g), exposed for 6 hours/day, 5 days/week for 3 weeks. The following results were seen:

– 100 ppm (425 $mg/m^3$): no symptoms of toxicity, the animals were in good condition throughout the exposure period. The organs appeared normal at autopsy.

– 300 ppm (1275 $mg/m^3$): a slight fall in the haemoglobin concentration and the haemoglobin content of individual erythrocytes ($Hb_e$) was seen on the third day of exposure. Histological examination of the organs produced no pathological findings.

– 1000 ppm (4250 $mg/m^3$): irritation of the nasal mucosa (sneezing, rhinitis) was seen initially. As the exposure continued there was decreased mobility and a reduced reaction to noise. The animals showed haemoglobinuria, porphyrinuria, reduced haemoglobin and $Hb_e$ (on day 4) and reticulocytosis. At the end of exposure, the blood and urine parameters had returned to normal. The organs appeared normal at autopsy and when examined histologically.

In a further subacute inhalation exposure study, groups of ten male and ten female rats were exposed to 0, 150 (638), 450 (1913) or 900 (3825) ppm ($mg/m^3$ air) for 6 hours daily, 5 days per week for 4 weeks. Body weight, food intake, and haematological, biochemical and urinary parameters were investigated, together with measurement of organ weight and macroscopic and microscopic examination of the organs. The actual concentrations of IPEGE were 142 (603), 441 (1874) and 891 (3787) ppm ($mg/m^3$ air). Body weight gain and food intake were not found to be affected. Haematological investigation revealed reductions in the haemoglobin concentration and in the number of erythrocytes in all groups, and an increase in the number of reticulocytes. The haematocrit level was reduced in both sexes in the medium and high concentration groups. In addition, biochemical tests revealed higher bilirubin levels after exposure to the highest concentration. Rats in the medium and high dose groups showed decreased urinary pH levels and a statistically significant increase in the absolute and relative spleen weight. Macroscopic evaluation of the internal organs revealed no abnormalities, but histopathological examination revealed treatment-related effects in the spleens of all animals (extramedullary haematopoiesis and accumulation of brown pigment). The authors concluded that these findings were indicative of haemolytic anaemia in all test groups. The no-effect-level in this study was assumed to be below 150 ppm (638 mg/m$^3$ air) in rats (CIVO-TNO, 1987a).

As the previous study did not permit a no-effect-level to be determined for IPEGE, a further 28-day inhalation study was conducted in rats. The animals were exposed to concentrations of 0, 10 (42.5), 30 (127.5) or 100 ppm (425 mg/m$^3$ air) for 6 hours daily, 5 days per week. Additional groups of five animals were used for a recovery period of 14 days. Body weight, haematological parameters, spleen weight and macroscopic and histopathological effects were assessed. The concentrations determined analytically during exposure corresponded to the nominal concentrations. No changes were seen in behaviour, condition or weight gain. Haematological investigation revealed a decrease in the haemoglobin concentration in females of the highest dose group, accompanied by a slight decrease in the number of erythrocytes and the haematocrit level and an increase in the average corpuscular volume. All these effects were reversed by the end of the recovery period. Spleen weight was normal, and macroscopic and microscopic examination of the spleen revealed no effects. A no-effect-level of 30 ppm (127.5 mg/m$^3$ air) was therefore established for repeated inhalation exposure in rats (CIVO-TNO, 1988a).

## 7.3 Skin and mucous membrane effects

In a skin irritation test on the clipped abdomen of the rabbit (0.01 ml IPEGE, uncovered, observation after 24 hours) the chemical was classified as a low-grade irritant (grade 3 on a 10-point scale; no further information; Smyth et al., 1969).

On instillation into rabbits' eyes, 0.005 ml IPEGE caused severe damage to the cornea (grade 5 on a 10-point scale; no further information; Smyth et al., 1969).

## 7.4 Sensitization

No information available.

7.5 Subchronic and chronic toxicity

Rats (age, strain and number not given) were exposed by inhalation to IPEGE at concentrations of 2.4 or 7.2 ppm (10 or 30 $mg/m^3$ air) for 3 months. They showed impaired function of the liver and kidney parenchyma (not described in detail), together with weight loss and reductions in the haemoglobin concentration and blood sugar levels. The authors suggested a no-effect-level of 0.72 ppm (3 $mg/m^3$ air; Lykova et al., 1976), but the study was inadequately conducted and evaluated.

7.6 Genotoxicity

No information available.

7.7 Carcinogenicity

No information available.

7.8 Reproductive toxicity

Female Wistar rats (13 weeks old, body weight 184–235 g) were exposed by inhalation to 50 (213), 150 (638) or 450 (1913) ppm ($mg/m^3$ air) IPEGE for 6 hours per day on days 6 to 15 of pregnancy. The dams exposed at the medium and high concentrations had haematuria. Haematological investigation (on days 8 and 16 of pregnancy) revealed decreases in the erythrocyte count, the haemoglobin concentration and the haematocrit level in the rats of the high exposure group and, to a lesser extent, in those exposed to the middle concentration. After treatment had ended (day 16 of pregnancy) a compensatory effect was observed (increases in the number of reticulocytes, the average corpuscular volume and the cell haemoglobin content). The fertility index of the dams was 87.5–92.5 and the gestation index was 100 in all groups. From days 6 to 10 of pregnancy, the rats in the middle and high concentration groups showed significant weight loss ($p<0.01$), and those in the low-dose group showed a significant reduction in body-weight gain ($p<0.05$) compared with the control group. In the second part of the treatment period a dose-dependent increase in body-weight gain was seen in all groups. The chemical did not affect the macroscopic appearance of the internal organs, the organ weights or the litter size of the dams. The highest concentration led to a significant increase in the number of immature foetuses. No teratogenic effect was observed in any of the dose groups. The no-effect-level for embryotoxicity was 150 ppm (CIVO-TNO, 1987b).

In a further embryotoxicity study, female New Zealand rabbits (6 months old, body weight 3561–4402 g) were exposed to concentrations of 20, 90 or 400 ppm IPEGE (corresponding to 85, 383 or 1700 mg/m$^3$ air) by inhalation for 6 hours daily on days 6 to 18 of pregnancy. The treatment did not give rise to any symptoms of toxicity. The fertility index was 83.3–100 and the gestation index was 100 in all groups. Maternal bodyweight gain was slightly reduced in the highest exposure group. The food intake of this group was significantly reduced during the observation period. Haematological investigation revealed decreases in the erythrocyte count, the haemoglobin concentration and the haematocrit level. Correlating with this, the mean corpuscular volume, the mean corpuscular haemoglobin content of the erythrocytes and the number of reticulocytes were increased in the highest exposure group. Macroscopic examination of the dams revealed no treatment-related effects. The average placental and foetal weights were slightly reduced at the top dose, and macroscopic evaluation of the foetuses showed an increased number of immature foetuses in this group. No foetotoxic effects were observed at the lower concentrations. No teratogenic effects were evident in any of the exposure groups. The no-effect-level with regard to foetotoxicity was 90 ppm (CIVO-TNO, 1988b).

In an acute study, male rats were exposed to a saturated vapour of IPEGE for 3 hours. Examination of the testes at the end of the 14-day observation period (on the 15th day after exposure) provided no indication of damage (no further details; Doe, 1984; Samuels et al. 1984).

The teratogenic effect of IPEGE was studied in two *in vitro* tests (not validated) in human mesenchymal embryo cells and V79 cells from the Chinese hamster, based on cell-to-cell communication after radioactive labelling. The authors put forward the hypothesis that the inhibition of cell-to-cell communication, possibly through gap junctions, resulted in a teratogenic effect because important signals for embryonic development were not being conveyed in the early cell phase (Welsch and Stedman, 1984a, b). The results of these studies and their interpretation are questionable.

## 7.9 Effects on the immune system

No information available.

## 7.10 Neurotoxicity

No information available.

7.11 Other effects

Carpenter et al., (1956) tested the osmotic resistance of erythrocytes in groups of six female rats (strain not specified) exposed for 4 hours to various vapour concentrations of IPEGE. The osmotic resistance was determined before and immediately after exposure. At concentrations of 32–62 ppm (136–264 mg/m$^3$ air), decreased osmotic resistance and marked haemolysis occurred.

## 8. Experience in humans

The odour threshold in humans is reported to be 0.768 ppm (3.2 mg/m$^3$ air). However, a lower level (0.6 ppm ≈ 2.5 mg/m$^3$ air) was found to influence the bioelectrical activity of the brain (no further details; Lykova et al., 1976).

## References

CIVO-TNO (CIVO-Toxicology and Nutrition TNO, Netherland)
A subacute (28-day) inhalation toxicity study of isopropyl ethylene glycol ether in rats
Report no. V85.434/241372 (1987a)
commissioned by BG Chemie

CIVO-TNO (CIVO-Toxicology and Nutrition TNO, Netherland)
Inhalation embryotoxicity/teratogenicity study with isopropyl ethylene glycol ether in rats
Report no V85.416/251371 (1987b)
commissioned by BG Chemie

CIVO-TNO (CIVO-Toxicology and Nutrition TNO, Netherland)
A subacute (28-day) inhalation toxicity study of isopropyl ethylene glycol ether followed by a 14-day recovery period in rats
Report no. V87.299/260985 (1988a)
commissioned by BG Chemie

CIVO-TNO (CIVO-Toxicology and Nutrition TNO, Netherland)
Inhalation embryotoxicity/teratogenicity study with isopropyl ethylene glycol ether in New Zealand white rabbits
Report no. V88.222 (1988b)
commissioned by BG Chemie

Clayton, G.D., Clayton, F.E. (eds.)
Patty's Industrial Hygiene and Toxicology
3rd ed., Vol. 2C, p. 3909
John Wiley and Sons, New York (1982)

Carpenter, C.P., Pozzani, U.C., Weil, C.S., Nair, J.S., Keck, G.A., Smith, H.F.
The toxicity of butyl cellosolve solvent
Arch. Ind. Health, 14, 114–131 (1956)

Doe, J.E.
Further studies on the toxicology of the glycol ethers with emphasis on rapid screening and hazard assessment
Environ. Health Perspect., 57, 199–206 (1984)

Gage, J.C.
The subacute inhalation toxicity of 109 industrial chemicals
Brit. J. Ind. Med., 27, 1–18 (1970)

Hutson, D.H., Pickering, B.A.
The metabolism of isopropyl oxitol in rat and dog
Xenobiotica, 1, 105–114 (1971)

Lykova, A.S., Shachkov, M.A., Mitrofanova, A.B., Davydova, M.P., Saparmamedov, E.S.
Data for the hygienic standardization of monoisopropyl and monobutyl ethers of ethyleneglycol in the atmosphere
Gig. Sanit., 11, 7–11 (1976)

Samuels, D.M., Doe, J.E., Tinston, D.J.
The effects on the rat testis of single inhalation exposure to ethylene glycol monoalkyl ethers, in particular ethylene glycol monomethyl ether
Arch. Toxicol., Suppl. 7, 167–170 (1984)

Saparmamedov, E.S.
Toxicity of some ethylene glycol ethers
Zdravookhr. Turkm., 18, 26–31 (1974)

Smyth, H.F., Carpenter, C.P., Weil, C., Pozzani, U.C., Striegel, J.A., Nycum, J.S.
Range-finding toxicity data: List VII
Am. Ind. Hyg. Assoc. J., 30, 470–476 (1969)

Weast, R.C. (ed.)
CRC-Handbook of Chemistry and Physics
62nd ed., C-296
CRC-Press, Boca Raton, Florida (1981/82)

Welsch, F., Stedman, D.B.
Inhibition of metabolic cooperation between Chinese hamster V 79 cells by structurally diverse teratogens
Teratogenesis Carcinog. Mutagen., 4, 285–301 (1984a)

Welsch, F., Stedman, D.B.
Inhibition of intercellular communication between normal human embryonal palatal mesenchyme cells by teratogenic glycol ethers
Environ. Health Perspect., 57, 125–133 (1984b)

Werner, H.W., Mitchell, J.L., Miller, J.W., von Oettingen, W.F.
The acute toxicity of vapors of several monoalkyl ethers of ethylene glycol
J. Ind. Hyg. Toxicol., 25, 157–163 (1943a)

Werner, H.W., Nawrocki, C.U., Mitchell, J.L., Miller, J.W., von Oettingen, W.F.
Effects of repeated exposures of rats to vapors of monoalkylethyleneglycolethers
J. Ind. Hyg. Toxicol., 25, 374–379 (1943b)

# Phenylglycidyl ether

## 1. Summary and assessment

On oral administration, phenylglycidyl ether (PGE) is rapidly adsorbed, metabolised in the liver and excreted in the urine. 2-Hydroxy-3-phenoxy propionic acid and N-acetyl-S(2-hydroxy-3-phenoxypropyl)-L-cysteine have been chromatographically detected as metabolites in the urine.

The acute toxicity of PGE is low in rats, mice and rabbits both orally and dermally ($LD_{50}$ oral, 1.4–4.2 g/kg body weight, dermal 2.16–2.99 g/kg body weight). PGE is toxic on acute inhalation exposure ($LC_{50}$ >100–323 ppm). Dyspnoea and depression of the central nervous system occur on oral administration to rats and mice. On inhalation by rats, dyspnoea, eye-watering, salivation, rhinitis, irritation of the lungs and interstitial pneumonia are observed.

Repeated inhalation of PGE causes decreased weight gain, atrophic changes to various organs (e.g. degeneration of the seminiferous tubules) and chronic catarrhal tracheitis. One case of inflammatory skin irritation has been seen.

Application of PGE to rabbits' skin causes slight skin irritation. A moderate irritant effect occurs in rabbits' eyes. PGE is a skin sensitizer, both in animal studies and in humans.

PGE induces dose-related mutations in *Salmonella typhimurium* strains TA 100 and TA 1535, in *Escherichia coli* WP2uvrA and in *Klebsiella pneumonia,* with and without the addition of a metabolising system. PGE is positive in the host-mediated assay. It does not induce mutations at either toxic or non-toxic doses in CHO-cells. PGE does not cause chromosome aberrations in vitro or micronucleus-formation in mice treated in vivo. Moreover, there is no indication of a dominant lethal effect in rats. DNA-binding does not occur in vitro. Oral administration of PGE to mice has no inhibitory effect on testicular DNA synthesis.

Chronic inhalation of 12 ppm PGE for 24 months leads to the development of nasal tumours in male and female rats. No treatment-related pathological changes are seen on exposure to 1 or 12 ppm for 12 months. PGE does not significantly increases SA7 virus transformation in primary hamster embryo cells, but does cause cell transformation of secondary hamster embryo cells.

In a two-generation study on reproductive toxicity, the chemical has no effect on weight gain and fertility of the $F_0$-males, on the number of offspring and their survival rate or on lactation. A teratogenicity study in rats has not given indication of an embryotoxic or teratogenic effect of PGE.

PGE is a reactive alkylating agent. PGE causes skin irritation and allergic reactions in man. Based on the available carcinogenicity studies, PGE is justifiably suspected to have a carcinogenic potential. Since 1984 it has been classified in section IIIB of the German list of MAK-values.

## 2. Name of substance

| | | |
|---|---|---|
| 2.1 | Usual-name | Phenylglycidyl ether |
| 2.2 | IUPAC-name | 1,2-Epoxy-3-phenoxy-propane |
| 2.3 | CAS-No. | 122-60-1 |

## 3. Synonyms, common and trade names

Phenoxymethyloxirane
2,3-Epoxypropylphenyl ether
Glycidyl phenyl ether
PGE
Phenoxypropene oxide

## 4. Structural and molecular formulae

4.1 Structural formula

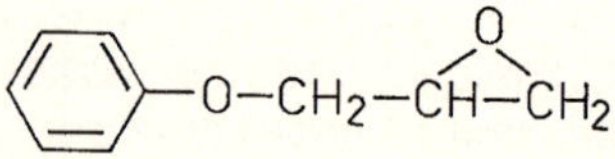


4.2 Molecular formula $C_9H_{10}O_2$

## 5. Physical and chemical properties

| | |
|---|---|
| 5.1 Molecular mass, g/mol | 150.17 |
| 5.2 Melting point, °C | 3.5 (Clayton and Clayton, 1981) |
| 5.3 Boiling point, °C | 245 (Clayton and Clayton, 1981) |
| 5.4 Vapour pressure, hPa | 0.013 (at 20 °C) (Clayton and Clayton, 1981) |
| 5.5 Density, g/cm$^3$ | 1.1092 (at 20 °C) (Clayton and Clayton, 1981) |
| 5.6 Solubility in water | 0.24% (Clayton and Clayton, 1981) |
| 5.7 Solubility in organic solvents | good in acetone and toluene<br>12.9% in octane<br>(Clayton and Clayton, 1981) |
| 5.8 Solubility in fat | No information available |
| 5.9 pH-value | – |
| 5.10 Conversion factor | 1 ppm $\hat{=}$ 6.13 mg/m$^3$<br>1 mg/m$^3$ $\hat{=}$ 0.16 ppm<br>(at 25 °C and 1013 hPa) |

## 6. Uses

As a stabilizer (acid acceptor) in halogenated compounds and as a so-called reactive diluent to reduce the viscosity of epoxy resins (Clayton and Clayton, 1981).

## 7. Experimental results

7.1 Toxicokinetics and metabolism

The metabolism of Phenyl glycidyl ether (PGE) was studied in Wistar rats (initial weight 250–300 g) and New Zealand white rabbits (initial weight 3.5–4 kg; sex and number of animals per group and dose of PGE not specified). PGE was administered as an aqueous suspension by stomach tube. The urine of the animals was collected 24 hours before administration and then at 24-hour intervals until no further excretion of metabolites could be detected. Chromatographic studies showed that rats and rabbits treated with PGE excrete

2-hydroxy-3-phenoxypropionic acid and N-acetyl-S-(2-hydroxy-3-phenoxypropyl)-L-cysteine as metabolites (James et al., 1978).

In vitro studies (hollow fibre technique, S9-mix from rat liver homogenate) revealed that the metabolism proceeds by means of conjugation aided by glutathione-S-alkyltransferase (Tsikas and Brunner, 1989; De Moerloose et al., 1983).

Acute dermal treatment of rats and rabbits with PGE showed that the substance is well adsorbed through the skin (dose not specified). Rates of absorption of 13.5 mg/m$^2$/hour for rats and 4.2 mg/m$^2$/hour for rabbits were measured (Czajkowska and Stetkiewicz, 1972).

7.2 Acute and subacute toxicity

Groups of 5 male Carworth-Wistar rats (initial weight 90–120 g) were given single doses of PGE in logarithmically increasing amounts. The observation period ws 14 days. An $LD_{50}$ value of 4.26 g/kg (3.90–4.66 g/kg) was determined (no further details; Smyth et al., 1984).

The oral $LD_{50}$ has also been investigated in male Long Evans rats (initial weight 89–150 g) and male Webster mice (initial weight 16–32 g). The groups were comprised of 5 rats and 6 mice, which were given neat PGE by stomach tube. The observation period was 10 days. The $LD_{50}$ was 3.85 (3.11–4.78) g/kg for rats and 1.4 (1.18–1.67) g/kg for mice. Administration of the chemical led to dyspnoea and depression of the central nervous system with impaired co-ordination, ataxia, reduced motor activity and coma. In the animals that survived exposure to PGE, the depressive effect was reversible, and increased activity of the central nervous system ensued (hypersensitivity to noise, muscle tremors, quivering; Hine et al., 1956).

In another study, a single dose of PGE was given to white Wistar rats (weight 250–350 g) by stomach tube. The observation period was 14 days. An $LD_{50}$ of 2.6 g/kg body weight was determined. Histopathological examination of the livers of the animals that died revealed nodule formation and necrosis of the liver parenchyma (Czajkowska and Stetkiewicz, 1972).

$LC_{50}$ values exceeding 100 ppm were determined for male Webster mice (initial weight 20–28 g; 5 to 6 mice per group; exposure time 4 hours) and for male Long-Evans rats (initial weight 110–140 g; 6 rats per group; exposure time 8 hours). Concentrations above 100 ppm PGE in the inhaled air could not be administered for technical reasons. The observation period was 10 days. Dyspnoea, watering eyes, salivation, rhinitis and aerophagy were observed in the animals. At post-mortem, marked irritation of the lung accompanied by acute interstitial pneumonia was seen. This was confirmed by histological examination (Hine et al., 1956).

Terrill and Lee (1977) reported an approximate lethal dose by inhalation of ca. 323 ppm (vapour-aerosol mixture) in male Sprague-Dawley rats (initial weight 250–260 g; 6 rats per group; exposure time 4 hours). Rats that survived lower exposure concentrations showed weight loss and pronounced irritation of the scrotum during the 14-day observation period.

A single application of PGE was made to the skin of white Wistar rats. The observation period was 14 days. A dermal $LD_{50}$ value of 2.16 g/kg body weight was determined. Histopathological examination of the skin 18 hours after treatment revealed necrosis, epithelial exfoliation and oedema. After 14 days, scar formation, acanthosis and swelling of the dermis were seen (Czajkowska and Stetkiewicz, 1972).

The dermal $LD_{50}$ was determined in rabbits (strain and sex not specified; initial weight 2.0–2.5 kg). Neat PGE was applied for 7 hours under cover to the clipped dorsal skin. An $LD_{50}$ of 2.99 (1.47–6.10) g/kg was reported (Hine et al., 1956).

In male New Zealand rabbits (initial weight 2.5–3.5 kg; 4 rabbits per group) a dermal $LD_{50}$ for PGE of 1.50 (1.07–2.10) g/kg was determined. The chemical was applied to the clipped dorsal skin (ca. one tenth of the surface area of the body), and contact was maintained under a plastic film for 24 hours. The observation period was 14 days (Smyth et al., 1954).

A subcutaneous $LD_{50}$ for PGE of 760 mg/kg was determined in an investigation involving a total of 60 mice (no further details; Söllner and Irrgang, 1965).

Intramuscular injection of 400 mg PGE/kg into rats on 3 consecutive days led to an increase in the number of leukocytes in the blood (no further details; Lane, 1980).

Six male Sprague-Dawley rats (initial weight 250–260 g) were exposed to 29 ppm PGE (vapour-aerosol mixture) by inhalation for 4 hours a day, 5 days a week for 2 weeks (i.e. 10 periods of exposure). Six rats served as untreated controls. All of the rats were weighed daily and examined for clinical symptoms. After 2 weeks, 3 rats each from the control and treatment groups were killed, the remaining rats being killed after a 2-week observation period. All of the rats were subjected to histological examination. Weight gain in the PGE-treated rats was reduced. In addition, there were atrophic changes to the kidneys, liver, spleen, thymus and testes, as well as chronic catarrhal tracheitis (Terrill and Lee, 1977).

Inhalation exposure of rats (8 per group) to 1.75, 5.84 and 11.2 ppm PGE for 6 hours/day on 19 consecutive days led to localized degeneration of the seminiferous tubules (1 rat in the 1.75 ppm group, 1 in the 5.84 ppm group, and 3 in the 11.2 ppm group; no further details; Lane, 1980).

## 7.3 Skin and mucous membrane effects

To investigate the irritant effect of PGE, 0.5 ml of the neat substance was applied to the clipped dorsal skin of albino rabbits under cover (initial weight of the rabbits 2–3 kg, sex not specified). The rabbits were then immobilized for 24 hours. At this point, and after 72 hours, the application site was examined and the severity of irritancy evaluated. PGE caused slight irritation. In a further study the irritant effect of PGE (over 24 hours) on the shaved skin of 5 albino rabbits was reported as 5 on a scale from 1 to 10 (no further details; Hine et al., 1956).

Neat PGE (0.5 ml) was applied with a gauze patch to the shaved and abraded skin of 3 albino rabbits. The treatment was occlusive and exposure was for 24 hours. The Draize scoring system was used (to evaluate reddening and swelling) 24 and 72 hours after application. PGE caused severe skin irritation and burns (Reichhold Chemicals, 1978).

In a further skin irritation study, 5 to 10 ml neat PGE was applied to the clipped and abraded skin of 6 albino rabbits and covered with a gauze patch. The patches were secured with 2 strips of adhesive tape and a strip of rubber adhesive tape was wrapped around the body of the rabbit. The rabbits were restrained for 24 hours, then the patches were removed and the treatment site was rinsed. The effects were evaluated directly after the patch was removed and again 72 hours later. Examination revealed effects ranging from considerable localized erythema to moderate diffuse erythema. In some places the skin was leathery with peripheral erythema formation (Reichhold Chemicals, 1978).

To investigate the irritant effect in rabbits' eyes 0.1 ml neat PGE was instilled into one eye, while the other eye served as a control. Irritancy was assessed after 1, 24 and 48 hours and was classified by the authors as slight (Hine et al., 1956).

Smyth et al. (1954) classified the irritant effect of PGE on rabbits' eyes as grade 2 on a scale from 1 to 10 (no further information).

7.4 Sensitization

The substance (5% in ethanol) was rubbed onto the skin of 10 guinea-pigs daily for 34 days. A challenge was then carried out with a 1% solution of PGE in ethanol. PGE had a sensitizing effect on guinea-pig skin (Rudzki and Krajewska, 1979).

The sensitization potential of PGE was investigated in albino guinea-pigs (Hartley strain, body weight 350–502 g) by means of the Bühler Patch Method. Twenty animals were used for the treatment group and 10 for the control. For induction, the guinea-pigs were treated with a 5% PGE solution in 80% ethanol, 3 times at weekly intervals. After an interval of 2 weeks, a challenge was carried out with a 0.5% solution of PGE in acetone. Evaluations were made 24 and 48 hours after the application. The results showed that PGE had a sensitizing effect in guinea-pigs (Reichhold Chemicals, 1978).

In a further sensitization study (ear-flank test based on the method of Turk and Stone, 1963), 0.1 ml of a 10% solution of PGE in olive oil was painted onto the outside of the ears of 6 albino guinea-pigs (Alderly Park strain, aged about 2 months) on 3 consecutive days. Seven days after the beginning of the study, 0.2 ml of a 10% solution of PGE in olive oil was applied to the clipped flank. The evaluation was carried out 24 hours later. A control group of 6 guinea-pigs was painted with 10% PGE in olive oil for the first time on day 7 of the study, and the site was similarly evaluated 24 hours after application. The results indicate that PGE has sensitization potential (Stevens, 1967).

As early as 1965 it was suggested that PGE was a potential sensitizer based on the results of a non-standardized patch test in guinea-pigs (Zschunke and Behrbohm, 1965).

7.5 Subchronic and chronic toxicity

In a 90-day inhalation study involving 63 exposures, 32 male and 32 female Sprague-Dawley rats (weight of the males 250–260 g and of the females 180–200 g) and 6 male beagles (weight 10–12 kg) were exposed to PGE (purity 99.6%) at concentrations of 0.1 (1.3 $\pm$ 0.5), 5 (5.0 $\pm$ 1.32) or 12 (11.8 $\pm$ 2.8) ppm for 6 hours daily, 5 days a week. The concentrations were measured hourly by means of UV analysis of impinger samples (sensitivity 1 ppm). The animals were examined every day for clinical symptoms and were weighed twice a week. On days 30, 60 and 90 of exposure and days 30, 60 and 90 of the observation period, blood and urine samples were taken for analysis from 10 male and 10 female rats per dose and from all of the dogs. Six rats of each sex per dose were killed on days 30, 60 and 90 of exposure and on the 28th day after the end of exposure for histopathological studies. Three dogs per dose group were killed after the last exposure and after the 90-day observation period. In both species haematological and clinical-chemical studies were carried out to determine the following parameters: serum glutamate-pyruvate transaminase (SGPT) activity, alkaline phosphatase (AP) activity, glucose levels, the numbers of red and white blood cells, packed cell volume and haemoglobin levels. In addition, the levels of urinary nitrogen, cholesterol, creatinine, the albumin/globulin ratio and protein levels were determined in dogs. In the urine of both rats and dogs, osmolarity, volume, colour, sediment, sugar, protein, blood and urobilinogen were analyzed. All animals were macroscopically examined at autopsy. The following organs were weighed: brain, heart, lungs, liver, kidneys, spleen, thyroid gland, pituitary gland, adrenal glands, testes and ovaries. The relationship between organ and body weight was calculated. Microscopic examinations were made of the lungs, trachea, heart, aorta, spleen, bone marrow, lymph nodes, thorax, liver, stomach, duodenum, jejunum, ileum, caecum, colon, rectum, pancreas, kidneys, bladder, salivary glands, thyroid gland, adrenal glands, pituitary gland, thymus, testes, epididymides, prostate, ovaries, uterus, mammary glands, brain, spinal cord, eyes, sciatic nerve, muscle, gall bladder (dog) and skin. There were no treatment-related effects in the rats either during or after exposure except for significant hair loss, which occurred in both sexes in the 5 and 12 ppm dose groups from about day 45 of treatment. At the end of the 90-day exposure period, 10% of the males and 25% of the females in the two higher dose groups had bald patches, particularly on the head, neck and shoulders. Weight gain in rats and dogs was normal compared with controls. No deaths occurred before the end of the study. Analysis of the blood and urine and histopathological examination did not reveal any treatment-related effects. The rats that suffered hair loss also developed acanthosis, parakeratosis and inflammatory cell infiltration of the skin and hair follicles. Normal hair growth was impaired (Terrill and Lee, 1977; Terrill et al., 1982).

In a sub-chronic inhalation study, 10 male Long-Evans rats were exposed to 100 ppm PGE (nominal concentration) for 7 hours daily for 50 days. Ten animals were used as untreated controls. The rats were closely observed and were weighed once a week. At the end of the study, blood samples were taken for haemoglobin determination. The rats were dissected and macroscopically examined. The lungs, liver and kidneys were weighed and the ratio of organ weight to body weight was determined. Histological examinations were made of the brain, thymus, heart, stomach, intestines, pancreas, adrenal glands, testes and bladder. Weight gain and relative organ weights were the same in the treated animals and the controls. Only the haemoglobin value was significantly higher ($p<0.01$) in the PGE-exposed rats than in the controls (Hine et al., 1956).

PGE (0.2 ml neat) was applied 5 times a week to the clipped dorsal skin of 6 albino rabbits (sex unspecified). One hour after application, the substance was removed with a cloth moistened with acetone. On the 4th day of treatment the rabbits exhibited severe skin irritation (erythema, oedema). After the 5th application, the treatment was cut short; no observations were made with regard to systemic toxicity (Hine et al., 1956).

## 7.6 Genotoxicity

### 7.6.1 In vitro

PGE was tested in the Salmonella/microsome test in *Salmonella typhimurium* strains TA 98, TA 100, TA 1535, TA 1537 and TA 1538, with and without metabolic activation (S9-mix from rat liver, induced with Aroclor 1254). Doses of 0.5–500 µg/plate were used. PGE caused dose-dependent mutations in strains TA 100 and TA 1535 with and without the addition of a metabolizing system; no cytotoxic effects were seen at this dose range (Greene et al., 1979).

In a further study, doses of 0.035–3.33 µmol/plate were investigated in the Salmonella/microsome test in *Salmonella typhimurium* strains TA 98, TA 100, TA 1535 and TA 1537, with and without an activation system (S9-mix from rat liver; no further details). PGE proved to be a dose-dependent mutagen in strains TA 100 and TA 1535. PGE was not cytotoxic at the doses tested (Ivie et al., 1980).

Similarly, PGE induced dose-dependent mutations (0.033–0.666 µmol/plate) in *Salmonella typhimurium* strains TA 100 and TA 1535 in a study by Neau et al. (1982). The study was carried out without metabolic activation. No cytotoxic effects were seen at this dose range.

Seiler (1984) showed that PGE was a dose-dependent point mutagen in *Salmonella typhimurium* without the addition of a metabolizing system (dose range 50–1000 μg/plate). These results were confirmed in a comparable study (Rosman et al., 1988).

In a further study in *Salmonella typhimurium* strains TA 97, TA 98, TA 100 and TA 1535 with and without metabolic activation (Aroclor 1254-induced hamster and rat liver), PGE induced point mutations in strains TA 97, TA 100 and TA 1535 (Canter et al., 1986).

*Escherichia coli* WP2uvrA was used as an indicator organism to investigate the mutagenic activity of PGE (20–10,000 μmol). No metabolizing system was added. PGE was mutagenic in this study (Hemminki et al., 1980).

PGE had a dose-dependent mutagenic effect in a fluctuation test with *Klebsiella pneumoniae* at 4 concentrations (0.1 to 1 μmol/l; Voogd et al., 1981).

At doses ranging from 6.25 to 100 μg/ml, which extended into the toxic dose range, PGE did not induce any 6-thioguanine-resistant mutations in CHO (Chinese hamster ovary) cells, with or without the addition of S9-mix (from Aroclor 1254-induced rat liver) or with or without serum in the medium (Greene et al., 1979).

Concentrations of 8 or 25 μg PGE/ml were tested in a chromosome aberration assay in Chinese hamster cells (CHO-K1-cells). After the cells had been incubated for 24 hours, the test substance (dissolved in DMSO) was added, and incubation continued for a further 6 to 24 hours. The cells were then examined. PGE did not induce chromosomal aberrations (Seiler, 1984).

PGE was negative in an in vitro study which measured DNA-binding to Ehrlich-ascites cells (DNA-cell binding test; Kubinski et al., 1981).

7.6.2 In vivo

PGE was also tested in a host-mediated assay, in C57B1/6×$C_3$H mice which had been inoculated intraperitoneally with *Salmonella typhimurium* TA 1535. Immediately after inoculation the mice were given 2500 mg PGE/kg orally or by intramuscular or intraperitoneal injection and 3 hours later they were killed. PGE was active in 2 out of 5 mice after oral treatment and in 1 out of 5 mice after intramuscular administration. It was inactive after intraperitoneal administration (Greene et al., 1979).

A micronucleus test was carried out in male and female mice (ICR strain, weight 25 g). The mice were given the test substance once orally in polyethylene glycol 400 at doses of 400, 500, 800 or 1000 mg/kg body weight. The mice were killed 24 hours after administration and their bone marrow was removed and processed. Fixing was carried out 24, 48 and 72 hours after administration. The bone marrow preparations were subsequently examined for the occurrence of micronuclei. PGE did not induce micronucleus-formation (Seiler, 1984).

A dominant lethal test was carried out in Sprague-Dawley rats (for description of study see Sect. 7.8). The parameters studied included the numbers of corpora lutea, implants and dead implants, pre- or post-implantation losses, the number of litters with early or late resorptions and the number of viable foetuses. There were no indications of a dominant lethal effect (Terrill et al., 1982).

Oral administration of PGE (500 mg/kg) to C57B1/6×$C_3H$ mice had no inhibitory effect on testicular DNA synthesis, as determined by $^3$H-thymidine-incorporation into DNA (Greene et al., 1979).

## 7.7 Carcinogenicity

The influence of PGE on SA7 virus transformation of primary hamster embryo cells (HEC) was studied at concentrations ranging from 1.6 to 1000 µg/ml. The transformation rate was significantly and dose-dependently increased by the addition of PGE at all concentrations that were not 100% toxic (1.6 to 40 µg/ml).

In tests on secondary hamster embryo cells, PGE had a cell-transforming effect at concentrations of 6.25 to 25 µg/ml. Concentrations of 50 and 100 µg/ml were cytotoxic (Greene et al., 1979).

Groups of 100 male and 100 female Sprague-Dawley rats were exposed to 0, 1 and 12 ppm PGE for 6 hours/day, five times a week for 2 years. After one year of treatment 10 males and 10 females from each group were killed and histopathologically examined. The surviving animals were killed after 2 years. The lungs, trachea, thyroid gland, parathyroid glands, pituitary gland, adrenal glands, testes and kidneys were histopathologically examined. The anterior and posterior nasal cavities were examined by light and electron microscopy. In the rats in the 12 ppm dose group, nasal tumours were first diagnosed after 621 days of exposure. The average latent period for tumours was 688 days. The incidence of nasal tumours was 9 out of 85 (11%) in the males and 4 out of 89 (4.4%) in the females. In the group exposed to 1 ppm no nasal tumours were observed in the 83 males or 88 females. A nasal tumour was seen in one of the 89 control males, but none were seen in the 87 control females. Histologically, the tumours were predominantly carcinomas, originating from the epidermis of the anterior nasal cavity. In addition, rhinitis was seen in the high-dose group (78%) along with squamous metaplasia of the nasal epithelium (72%; Lee et al., 1983).

7.8 Reproductive toxicity

In a two-generation study in male Sprague-Dawley rats, 4 groups of 8 male ($F_0$) rats (70 days old; initial weight about 360 g) were exposed to 0, 1, 5 or 12 ppm PGE for 6 hours per day on 19 consecutive days. Afterwards, at the beginning of each week, for a total of 6 weeks, groups of 3 untreated female rats ($F_0$) were put in a cage with each of the $F_0$-males for 5 days. Vaginal examinations were made daily, and after insemination had taken place the females were housed individually. After two recovery days the $F_0$-males were once again put with $F_0$-females, and this sequence continued until the end of the mating period. About half of the pregnant females were evaluated in a dominant lethal assay, whilst the remaining rats gave birth to their young ($F_1$-generation). The $F_1$-generation were weaned and mated within their treatment groups. The testes of the $F_0$-males were histologically examined. There was no significant difference compared with the controls with respect to the following parameters: weight gain, fertility of the $F_0$-males, number and survival rate of the offspring, and lactation behaviour (Terrill et al., 1982).

The same authors carried out a teratogenicity study, in which 100 pregnant Sprague-Dawley rats (initial weight about 200 g) were exposed to 0, 1, 5 and 12 ppm PGE for 6 hours a day on days 4 to 15 of pregnancy. The animals were killed on the 20th day of pregnancy. About two thirds of the foetuses from each litter were examined for skeletal anomalies while the remaining foetuses were checked for soft tissue anomalies. The weight and size of the foetuses was determined, along with the number of implantations, the number of live foetuses and the number of resorptions per litter. No embryotoxic or teratogenic effects were established for PGE (Terrill and Lee, 1977).

7.9 Effects on the immune system

No information available.

7.10 Neurotoxicity

No information available.

7.11 Other effects

In several studies on the pharmacological effects of PGE, the ability of PGE to alleviate spasms triggered in the intestines of guinea-pigs by barium chloride, acetyl choline and histamine was determined. PGE had a spasmolytic effect in all three cases. In a study of the muscle-relaxing effect of PGE, mice were placed in a rotating drum for 10 minutes, 30, 60 or 120 minutes after a subcutaneous injection with PGE, and the percentage of animals that fell out during this time was determined. The angle of inclination of the drum was 35°, and it revolved 8 times per minute. PGE acted as a muscle relaxant ($ED_{50}$ 30 minutes after injection: 430 mg/kg). The cataleptic activity of PGE was determined in the same animals after 30, 60 and 120 minutes. The $ED_{50}$ was given as 345 mg/kg, 30 minutes after injection. The effect of PGE on strychnine-induced convulsions was also measured. Two groups of 20 mice were given 1.33 or 0.65 mg strychnine/kg subcutaneously, with simultaneous subcutaneous administration of 100 mg PGE/kg. The incidence of convulsions in the mice was observed. The susceptibility to convulsions in PGE-treated mice was reduced compared with the controls, and the survival time increased (Söllner and Irrgang, 1965).

Fully-grown female Wistar rats were killed at intervals after PGE-administration, to determine the glutathione content of the liver. Approximately 30 minutes after PGE-administration (0.5 mmol/kg) there was a distinct fall in the glutathione content of the liver (after 1 hour, ca. 35% of the initial value); after 48 hours the level had returned to normal (James et al., 1978).

A study of the rate of alkylation by PGE was carried out by Hemminki et al. (1980). The nucleophiles used to determine the alkylation capacity were 4-(p-nitrobenzyl)pyridine (PGE concentration 0.286 μM) and deoxyguanosine (PGE concentration 0.1 M). PGE had an alkylating effect.

The alkylating effect of PGE in the p-nitrobenzylpyridine assay (according to Friedman and Bogner, 1961) was confirmed by Seiler (1984), the effect being dose-dependent in the dose range from 12.5 to 100 μg.

This effect was further confirmed in a comparable study by Rosman et al. (1988).

In an in vitro study in Ehrlich ascites carcinoma cells, it was shown that PGE inhibited the incorporation of $^{14}C$-labelled adenine and valine, indicating that PGE inhibits protein synthesis (Miko et al., 1978).

## 8. Experience in humans

Rudzki et al. (1983) reported 9 cases of occupational dermatitis following contact with PGE.

Hine et al. (1956) presented a total of 13 cases of dermatitis in people who had been exposed to PGE.

In a study of 58 patients who suffered from dermatitis and came into contact with PGE through their work, PGE was reported as the primary allergen in 9 people, based on the results of a patch test. Cross-reactions were observed between PGE and epoxy resins (Rudzki and Krajewska, 1979).

As early as 1975, Behrbohm and co-workers found a positive reaction in 2 cases in workers patch-tested with 1% PGE (Behrbohm et al., 1975).

Out of 74 workers who came into contact with a lubricating oil which contained PGE as a stabiliser, 16 developed a contact allergy. No further dermal symptoms occurred after the lubricating oil was changed for one which did not contain PGE (Hegyi and Jakubik, 1984).

Two out of 3 female employees who had developed an allergy to a two-component adhesive had a positive reaction to a patch test with PGE (Jolanki et al., 1987).

## 9. Threshold limit values

PGE has a MAK value of 1 ppm ($\hat{=}$ 6.13 $mg/m^3$), and is in category III B of the list of MAK values (DFG, 1984).

USA: Threshold limit value – TWA 1 ppm (ACGIH, 1986).

## References

ACGIH (American Conference of Governmental Industrial Hygenists, Inc.)
Threshold Limit Values Documentation
5th ed. (1986)

Behrbohm, P., Nehring, A., Nehring, P.
False negative tests with epoxy resin
Contact Dermatitis, 1, 267 (1975)

Canter, D.A., Zeiger, E., Haworth, S., Lawlor, T., Mortelmans, K., Speck, W.
Comparative mutagenicity of aliphatic epoxides in Salmonella
Mutat. Res., 172, 105–138 (1986)

Clayton, G.D., Clayton, F.E. (eds.)
Patty's Industrial Hygiene and Toxicology
John Wiley and Sons, New York, Vol. 2 A, p. 2213 (1981)

Czajkowska, T., Stetkiewicz, J.
Evaluation of acute toxicity of phenyl glycidyl ether with special regard to percutaneous absorption
Med. Pr., 23, 363–371 (1972)

De Moerloose, P., van den Eeckhout, E., Baeyens, W., de Bruyn, A., de Keukeleire, D.
Glutathionconjugatie als detoxificatiemechanisme van enkele alkeenepoxides
Verh. K. Acad. Geneeskd. Belg., 45, 491–508 (1983)

DFG (Deutsche Forschungsgemeinschaft)
Maximale Arbeitsplatzkonzentrationen 1984
Mitteilung XX der Senatskommission zur Prüfung gesundheitsschädlicher Arbeitsstoffe
Verlag Chemie, Weinheim (1984)

Friedman, O.M., Bogner, E.
Colorimetric estimation of nitrogen mustards in aqueous media
Anal. Chem., 33, 906–910 (1961)

Greene, E.J., Friedman, M.A., Sherrod, J.A., Salerno, A.J.
In vitro mutagenicity and cell transformation screening of phenylglycidyl ether
Mutat. Res., 67, 9–19 (1979)

Hegyi, E., Jakubik, A.
Skin damage from work with phenylglycidylether
Pracovni Lekarstvi, 36, 121–122 (1984)

Hemminki, K., Falck, K., Vainio, H.
Comparison of alkylation rates and mutagenicity of directly acting industrial and laboratory chemicals
Arch. Toxicol., 46, 277–285 (1980)

Hine, C.H., Kodama, J.K., Wellington, J.S., Dunlap, M.K., Anderson, H.H.
The toxicology of glycidol and some glycidyl ethers
Arch. Ind. Health, 14, 250–264 (1956)

Ivie, G.W., MacGregor, J.T., Hammock, B.D.
Mutagenicity of psoralen epoxides
Mutat. Res., 79, 73–77 (1980)

James, S.P., Pheasant, A.E., Solheim, E.
Metabolites of 1,2-epoxy-3-phenoxy- and 1,2-epoxy-3-(p-nitrophenoxy)propane
Xenobiotica, 8, 219–228 (1978)

Jolanki, R., Estlander, T., Kanerva, L.
Contact allergy to an epoxy reactive diluent: 1,4-butanediol diglycidyl ether
Contact Dermatitis, 16, 87–92 (1987)

Kubinski, H., Gutzke, G.E., Kubinski, Z.O.
DNA-cell-binding (DCB) assay for suspected carcinogens and mutagens
Mutat. Res., 89, 95–136 (1981)

Lane, J.M.
Glycidyl Ethers
Vert. Hum. Toxicol., 22, 99–101 (1980)

Lee, K.P., Schneider, P.W., Trochimowicz, H.J.
Morphologic expression of glandular differentiation in the epidermoid nasal carcinomas induced by phenylglycidyl ether inhalation
Am. J. Pathol., 111, 140–148 (1983)

Lee, K.P., Terrill, J.B., Henry, N.W.
Alopecia induced by inhalation exposure to phenyl glycidyl ether
J. Toxicol. Environ. Health, 3, 859–869 (1977)

Miko, M., Fancovic, K., Bakayova, T.
Effects of industrial epoxides on the metabolism of Ehrlich ascites carcinoma cells in vitro
Int. Cong. Ser. Excerpta Med., 440, 292–294 (1978)

Neau, S.H., Hooberman, B.H., Frantz, S.W., Sinsheimer, J.E.
Substituent effects on the mutagenicity of phenyl glycidyl ethers in Salmonella typhimurium
Mutat. Res., 93, 297–304 (1982)

Reichhold Chemicals, Inc.
Studies submitted under section 8(d) of the TSCA
U.S. Environmental Protection Agency, Office of Pesticides and Toxic Substances
8DHQ-0878-0007 (1978)

Rosman, L.B., Chakraborty, P.K., Messerly, E.A., Sinsheimer, J.E.
Mutagenicity of aromatic glycidyl ethers with *Salmonella*
Mutat. Res., 206, 115–125 (1988)

Rudzki, E., Krajewska, D.
Contact sensitivity of phenylglycidyl ether
Dermatosen, 27, 42–44 (1979)

Rudzki, E., Rebandel, P., Grzywa, Z., Jakiminska, B.
Dermatitis from phenyl glycidyl ether
Contact Dermatitis, 9, 90–91 (1983)

Seiler, J.P.
The mutagenicity of mono- and di-functional aromatic glycidyl compounds
Mutat. Res., 135, 159–167 (1984)

Smyth, H.F., Carpenter, C.P., Weil, C.S., Pozzani, U.C.
Range-finding toxicity data, List V
Arch. Ind. Hyg. Occup. Med., 10, 61–68 (1954)

Söllner, K., Irrgang, K.
Untersuchungen über die pharmakologische Wirkung aromatischer Glycidäther
Arzneimittelforschung, 15, 1355–1357 (1965)

Stevens, M.A.
Use of the albino guinea-pig to detect the skin-sensitizing ability of chemicals
Br. J. Ind. Med., 24, 189–202 (1967)

Terrill, J.B., Lee, K.P.
The inhalation toxicity of phenylglycidyl ether. 1. 90-day inhalation study
Toxicol. Appl. Pharmacol., 42, 263–269 (1977)

Terrill, J.B., Lee, K.P., Culik, R., Kennedy, G.L.
The inhalation toxicity of phenylglycidyl ether: reproduction, mutagenic, teratogenic and cytogenetic studies
Toxicol. Appl. Pharmacol., 64, 204–212 (1982)

Tsikas, D., Brunner, G.
Enzymatic detoxification using lipophilic hollow-fiber membranes: IV. glutathione conjugation reactions
Int. J. Artif. Organ., 12, 121–128 (1989)

Turk, J.L., Stone, S.H.
In cell-bound antibodies
Conference of the National Academy of Sciences
Eds.: Ames, B., Koprowski, H.
Wistar Institute Press, Philadelphia, 51–60 (1963)
Cited in: Stevens, 1967

Voogd, C.E., van der Stel, J.J., Jacobs, J.J.J.A.A.
The mutagenic action of aliphatic epoxides
Mutat. Res., 89, 269–282 (1981)

Zschunke, E., Behrbohm, P.
Ekzem durch Phenoxypropenoxyd und ähnliche Glyzidäther
Dermatol. Wochenschr., 19, 480–484 (1965)

# Thiram

## 1. Summary and assessment

A toxicological evaluation of thiram was produced by the DFG (MAK commission) in 1976. The results presented are incorporated here and are supplemented with more recent findings.

Thiram is absorbed from the intestinal tract and the respiratory tract. Distribution studies show that thiram is detectable in all tissues. It is partly excreted unchanged in the urine and faeces. It also forms dimethyldithiocarbamic acid in intermediary metabolism by cleavage of the sulphide bonds. At the same time carbon disulphide is formed and can be detected in the breath. It also forms tetramethyl thiourea in much smaller quantities. In the ruminant, microorganisms play a greater role in the metabolic breakdown of thiram. Carbon disulphide, hydrogen sulphide and dimethylamine are formed as end products.

Thiram is of low acute toxicity (rat, mouse oral $LD_{50}$ 800–4000 mg/kg body weight; rat, rabbit dermal >2000 mg/kg body weight; rat $LC_{50}$ 300–1000 mg/m$^3$ air). Toxic symptoms include impairment of the nervous system (ataxia, tremors), and, at higher doses, swelling of the abdomen and convulsions.

Similar symptoms are seen on repeated administration, with growth inhibition, weight loss, nervous disturbances and changes in blood morphology.

The compound has a slight irritant effect on the skin, but is severely irritating or corrosive to the mucous membranes with marked corneal atrophy.

A skin sensitizing effect has been described in guinea-pigs and rabbits. Studies involving intratracheal administration to guinea-pigs also indicate an immunological sensitization effect (immediate allergic reaction).

Thiram is mutagenic in the Salmonella/microsome test with and without the addition of a metabolising system. It is also positive in the DNA repair test and the Rec assay on *Bacillus subtilis*, and produces point mutations and aneuploidy in *Aspergillus nidulans*. Repair of DNA (UDS) in rat thymocytes does not take place. Both positive and negative results have been obtained in the SCE test in CHO-cells. In the HGPRT test the chemical is mutagenic to V79 cells at high concentrations but is not mutagenic to CHO cells at lower doses and with exogenous metabolism. In vivo studies (several micronucleus tests, bone marrow investigations on rats) indicate a clastogenic effect. An increase in recessive lethal mutations appears in the Drosophila test. Changes in sperm morphology have been observed in mice.

In carcinogenicity studies, no increase in tumours is observed after oral administration to mice or rats. A single subcutaneous injection similarly does not increase the tumour incidence. In two-year studies in rats a thyrogenic effect takes place (follicular hyperplasia, proliferation of the stroma, formation of follicular and trabecular adenomas).

There are clear indications of embryotoxicity and teratogenicity in mice, rats, hamsters and rabbits. Besides an increased incidence of resorptions in the middle and late phases of organogenesis, dose-dependent malformations such as cleft palate, micrognathia, kyphosis, wavy ribs and crooked phalanges also occur. Repeated oral or inhalation exposure of the dams leads to changes in the duration of oestrus (lengthening of dioestrus). In males exposed by inhalation (1 mg/m$^3$ air for 4 months), a decrease in the sperm count and degeneration of the spermatogenic epithelium is seen. No such effects occur after oral administration.

The effect of thiram in intermediary metabolism basically represents inhibition of various enzymes, cytochrome oxidase, succinate dehydrogenase, amylase, catalase, polyphenol oxidase, GOT and GPT and alcohol dehydrogenase (moderate) and aldehyde dehydrogenase (marked). As with all dithiocarbamates, the occurrence of Antabuse syndrome is to be expected on administration of thiram with alcoholic drinks. Thiram also has an antidiuretic effect (reduction of sodium and potassium excretion).

Increased motor activity is seen in the open-field test in young rats born to thiram-treated mothers.

Most of the effects seen in animal models (with regard to acute and chronic toxicity, irritant effects and skin sensitization acitivity) have also been observed in humans (acute: headaches, vomiting, heart arrhythmias, breathing difficulties, bronchitis, fall in blood pressure, liver damage, eosinophilia, lymphocytopenia, neutrocytopenia; chronic: functional disturbances of the liver and thyroid gland, atrophy of the respiratory tract, conjunctivitis, neuritis, jaundice and contact dermatitis). Contrary to the findings in animal studies, no indication of testicular damage or symptoms of paralysis have arisen in humans.

Increased incidences of toxicosis during pregnancy and of haemorrhaging after birth were seen in pregnant women who have had prolonged contact with thiram through their work in a seed-treatment plant.

A sperm toxicity test, two teratogenicity studies (oral) and three long-term studies (feeding studies in the rat, mouse and dog) are presently being carried out.

Thiram is of low acute toxicity, is slightly irritating to the skin but severely irritating or corrosive to the eyes and has a sensitization effect. The results of mutagenicity tests are partly contradictory, and mutagenic activity cannot be excluded. No carcinogenic activity has been established. On chronic administration, changes to the thyroid gland occur. Thiram has toxic effects on reproduction in several species. It inhibits a multitude of enzymes. With the exception of reproductive toxicity and symptoms of paralysis, comparable effects are seen in man.

Thiram may be contaminated with the carcinogen, dimethylnitrosamine, at various levels (between 4 and 800 µg/kg active chemical).

## 2. Name of substance

| | | |
|---|---|---|
| 2.1 | Usual name | Thiram |
| 2.2 | IUPAC-name | Bis-(dimethylthiocarbamoyl) disulphide |
| 2.3 | CAS-No. | 137-26-8 |

## 3. Synonyms, common and trade names

Arasan
Fernacol
Fernasan
Pomarsol
Pomasol
Tersan
Tetramethylthiuram disulphide
Thiosan
Thiotex
Thiuram
TMTD
Vulkacit Thiuram

## 4. Structural and molecular formulae

4.1 Structural formula

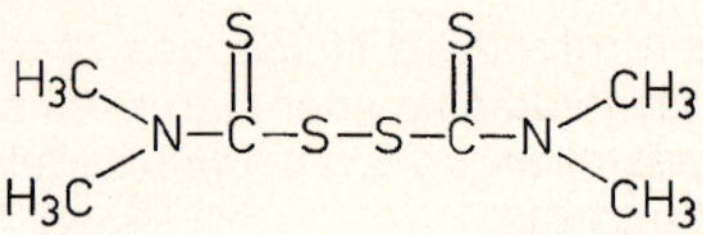

4.2 Molecular formula $C_6H_{12}N_2S_4$

## 5. Physical and chemical properties

| | | |
|---|---|---|
| 5.1 | Molecular mass, g/mol | 240.43 (Weast, 1982) |
| 5.2 | Melting point, °C | 155.6 (Weast, 1982) |
| 5.3 | Boiling point, °C | 129 (at 27 hPa) (Weast, 1982) |
| 5.4 | Vapour pressure, hPa | $<10^{-5}$ (at 20 °C) (IPS, 1982) |
| 5.5 | Density, $g/cm^3$ | 1.21 (at 20 °C) (Weast, 1982) |
| 5.6 | Solubility in water | 0.003 g/100 ml (at 20 °C) (IPS, 1982) |
| 5.7 | Solubility in organic solvents | Chloroform 230 g/l<br>Acetone 80 g/l<br>Ethanol <10 g/l<br>(Weast, 1982) |
| 5.8 | Solubility in fat | No information available |
| 5.9 | pH-value | – |
| 5.10 | Conversion factor | 1 ppm $\hat{=}$ 9.99 $mg/m^3$ air<br>1 $mg/m^3$ $\hat{=}$ 0.1 ppm<br>(at 25°C and 1013 hPa) |

## 6. Uses

Vulcanization accelerator, disinfectant for seeds, bacteriostatic agent, fungicide (Weast, 1982; Windholz, 1983; IPS, 1982; Worthing and Walker, 1983).

## 7. Experimental results

7.1 Toxicokinetics and metabolism

White male rats received a single intragastric dose of thiram corresponding to the $LD_{50}$. The animals were killed at various times and the thiram content of a number of tissues was determined (method not specified). Thiram was found in the blood and in the tissues of all of the organs 2 hours after administration. The maximum blood and tissue levels were seen on day 4; the highest concentrations were in the adrenal cortex (346 μg/g) and lower concentrations were seen in the thymus gland (179 μg/g), the spleen (73 μg/g), the blood 48 μg/g), the lungs (30 μg/g) and the urine (16 μg/ml). The lowest concentrations were found in muscle and brain tissues (Antonovich, 1973).

A similar distribution pattern was seen in an 8-month study in which thiram was administered (route unspecified) to rats at doses of 4, 2, 1 and 0.5 mg/kg. There was no correlation between the thiram concentration in the tissues and the dose level. The study demonstrated a prolonged elimination time for thiram. The half-life in the blood was 5.6 days, and that in the liver 5.5 days (Antonovich, 1973).

Thiram (dose not specified) was mainly excreted in the urine and the faeces. Dimethyldithiocarbamic acid was found in the blood, liver, spleen and lungs 2 days after a single administration of thiram. In addition, carbon disulphide ($CS_2$) was detected dose-dependently in the exhaled air. $CS_2$ was excreted for 4 days and reached a maximum on day 2. Tetramethylthiourea was detectable in the liver 6 days after administration. In mammals, thiram is reduced by glutathione to dithiocarbamate (no further details given; Antonovich and Vekshtein, 1970).

Dalvi and Deoras (1986) showed that, on intraperitoneal injection of thiram into rats, the formation of $CS_2$ as a metabolite was dose dependent. Male Sprague-Dawley rats (160–200 g) were given an intraperitoneal injection of 15, 30 or 60 mg thiram/kg body weight in corn oil, and the expiration of $CS_2$ was determined. The concentration of exhaled $CS_2$ increased with increasing dose.

In cannulated ruminants (cow, sheep), measurements in the stomach following oral administration of thiram-containing feed revealed that as a result of microbial activity (bacteria, protozoa) thiram was metabolized to $CS_2$, $H_2S$, and dimethylamine (Robbins and Katelic, 1961).

## 7.2 Acute and subacute toxicity

Thiram was of moderate acute oral toxicity ($LD_{50}$ rat 800–4000 mg/kg, mouse 1500–4000 mg/kg, hen 840 mg/kg, cat ca. 230 mg/kg, rabbit 210 mg/kg). The acute dermal toxicity was lower, with values of >1000 and 2000 mg/kg body weight in rats and rabbits, respectively. For single inhalation exposures, $LC_{50}$ values of >102 and between 300 and 1000 mg/$m^3$ air have been reported. The intraperitoneal $LD_{50}$ was more than 240 mg/kg in rats, and 250 mg/kg in mice (see Table 1). Observed symptoms included impaired breathing, ataxia, tremors, dyspnoea, abdominal distention and weight loss, with convulsions in the lethal dose range. The effects were delayed, occurring mainly on day 2 of the observation period. After acute inhalation exposure, irritation of the mucous membranes of the upper respiratory tract was also observed. No symptoms were seen on single dermal application (IPS, 1982; Izmerov, 1982; Dalvi, 1987; Lee et al., 1978; Antsiferov and Zhavoronkov, 1972; Brieger, 1947; see Table 1).

Male Wistar rats (weight ca. 78 g) were given 225, 300, 450, 600, 900 or 1200 ppm thiram daily in their feed for 30 days. On day

**Table 1.** Acute toxicity of thiram ($LD_{50}$/$LC_{50}$)

| Species | Sex | Route of Exposure | $LD_{50}$ (mg/kg) $LC_{50}$ (mg/$m^3$) | References |
|---|---|---|---|---|
| Rat | – | Oral | 800–3000 | IPS, 1982 |
| Rat | – | Oral | 400– 940 | Izmerov, 1982 |
| Rat | Male | Oral | 4000 | Lee et al., 1978 |
| Rat | Female | Oral | 1900 | Lee et al., 1978 |
| Mouse | – | Oral | 1500–2000 | IPS, 1982 |
| Mouse | – | Oral | 1250–2900 | Izmerov, 1982 |
| Mouse | Male | Oral | 4000 | Lee et al., 1978 |
| Mouse | Female | Oral | 3800 | Lee et al., 1978 |
| Rabbit | – | Oral | 210 | Antsiferov and Zhavoronkov, 1972 |
| Rabbit | – | Oral | 1200 | Brieger, 1947 |
| Rat | – | Inhalation | > 102 | Izmerov, 1982 |
| Rat | – | Inhalation | 300–1000 (4 hours) | IPS, 1982 |
| Rat | – | Dermal | >1000 | IPS, 1982 |
| Rabbit | – | Dermal | >2000 | Brieger, 1947 |
| Rat | Male | i.p. | > 240 | Dalvi, 1987 |
| Mouse | Male | i.p. | 250 | Izmerov, 1982 |

30, the animals were killed and organ weights were determined (liver, kidneys, heart, epididymal and perirenal fat, testes, seminal vesicle, tibia, adrenal glands and thyroid gland). Liver concentrations of lactate, pyruvate, β-hydroxybutyrate, acetoacetate, ATP and ADP were measured. There were dose-dependent decreases in food intake, body weight, perirenal fat and the weight of the kidneys, testes and epididymides as well as a decrease in the lactate-pyruvate ratio in the liver (Lowy et al., 1980).

Rats given 0.075 mg thiram/kg body weight orally for 30 or 45 days showed weight loss, nervous system effects and changes in blood biochemistry and composition (no further details; Stefan et al., 1972).

Rats (age, sex and strain not given), were exposed for 2 hours daily to 300 or 400 mg thiram/m$^3$ air for 15 days. Weight loss and central nervous system effects were seen (no further details; Vorob'eva and Mezentseva, 1962).

The same authors carried out an inhalation study on rabbits (age, strain and sex not specified), which were exposed to 1.9 mg thiram/m$^3$ air for 7 hours daily, 5 days/week for 5 weeks. The authors reported parenchymatous degeneration of the liver and kidneys with some necrosis, as well as irritation of the lungs (no further details; Vorob'eva and Mezentseva, 1962).

Groups of 50 male white leghorn chicks were given 30 or 60 mg thiram/kg in their feed. From week 2, ten chicks from each group were killed and their tibia were removed. The left tibia was used to determine bone ash, while a longitudinal section of the right tibia was examined for dyschondroplasia. The birds were kept under standard conditions. Thiram was found to cause tibial dyschondroplasia in chicks from the second week, the lesions increasing with the duration of treatment. In addition to effects on the bones, body weight was also reduced (Veltmann and Linton,1986).

Repeated daily oral administration of thiram in the feed of chickens (150 and 300 ppm), geese (150, 400 and 800 ppm) and turkeys (400 and 800 ppm) for 3 weeks led to weight loss and bone deformities (no further details; Waibl et al., 1957).

## 7.3 Skin and mucous membrane effects

In rabbits (strain, age and sex not specified) thiram was slightly irritating to the skin and strongly irritating or corrosive to the eyes, causing corneal necrosis (no further details; IPS, 1982).

## 7.4 Sensitization

Thiram caused contact allergy in guinea-pigs (no further details; Griepentrog, 1960).

Contact allergy was observed in albino rabbits following intracutaneous induction with 0.5% thiram and subsequent challenge with the same concentration. Hyperaemia, oedema, local haemorrhaging and ulceration of the skin were seen (Griepentrog, 1960).

In a further study, intratracheal induction followed by tracheal challenge provoked an anaphylactic reaction in guinea-pigs (no further details; Brusilovskiy and Fiallkovskiy, 1973).

## 7.5 Subchronic and chronic toxicity

Rats (number, age and sex not specified) were given thiram (Pomarsol, 80% WP) at concentrations of 0.5%, 0.03% or 0.01% in the daily feed (20 g) for 2–6 months. At the highest concentration epileptic-type convulsions were seen in two phases during the first and second months of the study but were not seen subsequently. Fairly uniform symptoms accompanied the convulsions, with rapidly increasing restlessness (during which the rats jumped and ran around their cages with increasing speed, frequently uttering sounds), followed by abrupt collapse with tonic-clonic spasms. The medium and low concentrations (0.03 and 0.01% thiram) did not produce any convulsive effects of this kind (Griepentrog, 1961).

Thiram was given to 20 young male rats (Charles-River) at concentrations of 0, 0.05, 0.1 or 0.25% in their feed for 13 weeks. At the end of the study, blood samples were taken for haematological and biochemical analyses. The liver, spleen, kidneys, adrenal glands, thyroid gland and gonads were weighed. After appropriate preparation, histopathological examinations were made of these organs and of the heart, lungs, salivary glands, pancreas, stomach, small intestine, bladder, genitals, diaphragm and muscle, ribs, pituitary gland and brain. A daily intake of 0.05% (30 mg/kg), 0.1% (58 mg/kg) or 0.25% (132 mg/kg) caused significant reductions in body weight and feed consumption in the male rats. One animal in the medium-dose group and 5 in the high-dose group died during the study. In the medium-dose group, a slight increase in blood urea was observed, and in the high-dose group there was an increase in the activity of aspartate aminotransferase (AST) and alanine aminotransferase (ALT). Moderate tubular degeneration in the testes and atypical spermatids in the epididymides were observed in the high-dose group (Lee et al., 1978).

Groups of 10 male and 10 female rats (Fischer-344) were given thiram at levels of 0.015, 0.03 or 0.06% in their feed for 13 weeks. Feed consumption and body weight were unaffected. Females in the high-dose group showed increased ALT, AST and lactate dehydrogenase (LDH) activities and slightly lower levels of cholinesterase. Slight cholangiolitis was seen in 5 female rats in the high-dose group, an effect that was not observed in the other groups. Male rats in the high-dose group had slightly increased AP activities, but no associated histopathological changes in the liver could be found. The authors concluded that the maximum tolerated dose of thiram was more than 0.06% in the feed (Kurata et al., 1980).

Thiram was administered to rats at a dose of 1 mg/kg in their drinking water (20 mg/l) for 6 months. This dose caused changes in the proportion of red blood cells and disturbances in liver and kidney function. A concentration of 0.04 mg/kg (0.8 mg/l) had no toxic effects. Combined exposure to 0.04 mg/kg in the drinking water and the maximum concentration of thiram in the air (not specified) led to functional changes in the haemoglobin level and the chloride content of the urine and to diuretic effects (Zhilenko, 1976).

Groups of 24 male and 24 female young rats (Charles-River) were given thiram in their feed at levels of 0.01, 0.04 or 0.1% for 80 weeks. A satellite group consisting of 4 rats of each sex from each dose group was killed and examined after 26 weeks. From week 14, the level in the feed was increased to 0.015, 0.06 or 0.15% respectively. A female in the high-dose group exhibited ataxia and atrophy of the muscles of the hind legs during week 20 and week 69. Six further females developed ataxia between weeks 39 and 80, showing an abnormal gait with dragging of the hind paws and the tail. The rats exhibited paralytic effects in the lumbar region and atrophy of the rear extremities. Towards the end of the study they were severely emaciated. Weight gain was retarded at all concentrations in males and at the middle and high concentrations in the females. Haematological and clinical-chemical investigations did not reveal any abnormalities. After 80 weeks, the relative weights of the thyroid gland and testes in the high-dose rats were increased, and the females showed increased relative weights of the liver, spleen, kidney, thyroid gland, ovaries and brain. In the medium-dose group the relative spleen weight was increased in the females. Histopathological examination revealed an increased incidence of fatty infiltration of the pancreas in the males. There was a slight increase in the number of metaplasias in the thyroid gland in both sexes in the highest dose group. No histopathologically identifiable changes were seen in the central or peripheral nervous system (Lee et al., 1978).

Significant changes in the peripheral blood (haemoglobin, erythrocytes, leukocytes and eosinophils), the liver and the nervous system were observed on subchronic exposure of rats and rabbits (age, origin and sex not specified) to 50 or 150 mg thiram/m$^3$ air for 1 hour daily over 4 months (no further details; Vorob'eva and Mezentseva, 1962; Vorob'eva and Kasparov, 1968).

## 7.6 Genotoxicity

The results of mutagenicity studies on thiram are summarized in Table 2. From this table it can be seen that thiram has a definite point-mutagenic effect both in vivo and in vitro, under various test conditions, and also causes chromosomal aberrations in vivo. It appears to have no effect on DNA-repair (UDS).

Khoroshilova et al. (1980) found an increased rate of chromosomal reorganisation in somatic and sex cells after repeated intragastric administration of 50 mg thiram/kg body weight for 2.5 months. A dose of 5 mg thiram/kg body weight had no such effect. No gonadotrophic effect was seen at either dose.

When thiram was incubated with nitrites at pH 3 or below, nitrosamine derivatives were formed which were similarly mutagenic in the Ames test (Egert and Greim, 1976; Andrews et al., 1980).

## 7.7 Carcinogenicity

In two series of tests, Sprague-Dawley rats of both sexes were given thiram at concentrations of 0.03% or 0.01% in their feed (ca. 20 g/day) for 2 years. In addition to thiram (Pomarsol), Lutiram and Polyram were also studied. Particular consideration was given to the observed effects on the thyroid gland, although the changes induced by each compound were presented and discussed together so that correlations are not possible. In addition to diffuse colloidal strumae, there were large-faced and trabecula adenomas and proliferating Langhans strumae. No carcinomas or metastases were observed. The author emphasized that such changes only developed after chronic intoxication (Griepentrog, 1962).

In a long-term study, mice (SPF-derived) were given thiram orally as the commercial preparation without further purification. The strains used were (C57B1/6xC3H/Anf)$F_1$ and (C57B1/6xAKR)$F_1$. The maximum tolerated dose at which no deaths occurred was determined in a preliminary study. Eighteen mice were used per strain and sex. In addition there was an untreated control group and a positive control group which received ethyl carbamide. Thiram was administered to the animals daily by stomach tube at a dose of 10 mg/kg, from 7 days of age to 4 weeks, and was subsequently administered in the food (26 ppm) up to the age of 18 months. At the end of the study a macroscopic examination of the animals and a histopathological examination of all organs was made. No increase in the tumour rate was found in this study (Innes et al., 1969).

In a carcinogenicity study, 30, 100 or 300 ppm thiram (99.6% pure) was given to groups of 50 male and 50 female NMRI mice (SPF derived, 7 weeks old) in their feed for 104 weeks. In addition, groups of 10 animals were used (same dosages) for haematological and clinical-chemical studies, with corresponding control groups. All animals which died during the study or which were killed at the end were macroscopically and histologically examined (brain, pituitary gland, eyes, salivary glands, larynx, thyroid gland, trachea, oesophagus, thymus, heart, aorta, lungs, stomach, liver, spleen, pancreas, mesentery, small and large intestine, kidneys, adrenal glands, bladder, mammary glands, ovaries, uterus, testes, epididymides, prostate gland, seminal vesicles, skeletal musculature, femurs, spinal column, sternum, skin, submandibular and mesenteric lymph nodes). With regard to appearance, behaviour and mortality, thiram had no effect in any of the dose groups. Feed consumption and body weight gain in the treated animals did not vary from that in the controls. Haematological values and urinary parameters for the treated groups and the controls were within the normal physiological range, as were the activities of glutamate-pyruvate transaminase (GPT) and alkaline phosphatase (AP). Fluctuations in organ weight in both sexes were neither substance- nor dose-related. Histopathological examination revealed no substance- or dose-dependent increase in the number of tumours in the treated animals compared with the controls (Brune, 1980).

Groups of 50 Fischer 344 rats (5 weeks old) were given thiram in their feed at concentrations of 0, 0.05 or 0.1% for 2 years (104 weeks). Body weight gain and mortality were recorded, as well as macroscopic and microscopic changes to the organs (no further details). The average body weight of the animals in the highest dose group (0.1%) was slightly reduced compared with the controls. The mortality was not significantly different between groups. Tumours were found in various organs of both males and females in all groups. There was no increase in the incidence of tumours compared with

**Table 2.** In vitro and in vivo mutagenicity tests with thiram

| Test system | Dose/ Solvent | Metabolic activation | Toxicity | Results (Reference) |
|---|---|---|---|---|
| In vitro | | | | |
| Salmonella/ microsome test TA 100, TA 98, TA 1535, TA 1537, TA 1538 | Up to 5000 μg/plate | No further details | Toxic from about 100 μg/plate | Mutagenic in TA 100 and weakly mutagenic in TA 1535 without metabolic activation. Not mutagenic in the remaining strains (Moriya et al., 1983) |
| Salmonella/ microsome test TA 100, TA 98, TA 1535, TA 1538 | 0, 50, 100, 150, 200 μg/ plate in DMSO | S9 mix from Aroclor-induced rat liver (Wistar) | Toxic from about 150 μg/plate | Dose-dependent mutagen in TA 100 and TA 1535 without metabolic activation. Decrease in mutagenicity with metabolic activation. Mutagenic in TA 1538 and TA 98 with metabolic activation (Zdzienicka et al., 1979) |

| | | | | |
|---|---|---|---|---|
| Salmonella/ microsome test TA 98, TA 100, TA 1535, TA 1537, TA 1538 | Not specified | S9 mix from Aroclor-induced rat liver (Sprague-Dawley) | Not specified | Mutagenic in TA 1535 and TA 100 without metabolic activation; questionable in the other strains (Hedenstedt et al., 1979) |
| Salmonella/ microsome test TA 98, TA 100, TA 1535, TA 1537, TA 1538 | Not specified | S9 mix from Aroclor-induced rat liver (Sprague-Dawley) | Not specified | Mutagenic in TA 98, TA 100 and TA 1535 from 5 μg/plate without metabolic activation. Additional increase in the number of revertants with metabolic activation (Rannug et al., 1984) |
| Salmonella/ microsome test TA 98, TA 100 | Not specified | Not specified | Not specified | Mutagenic in TA 100 (Kawachi et al., 1980) |
| Salmonella/ microsome test TA 1535, TA 1537, TA 1538, TA 98, TA 100 | Not specified | Not specified | Not specified | Mutagenic in TA 100 (Moriya et al., 1978) |

**Table 2** (continued)

| Test system | Dose/ Solvent | Metabolic activation | Toxicity | Results (Reference) |
|---|---|---|---|---|
| Induction of prophages in *Escherichia coli* | 0.1–10 µg in DMSO | S9 mix from Aroclor-induced rat liver (Wistar) | Not specified | No induction of prophages without S9 mix, slight induction of prophages with S9 mix (up to 55%) (Zdzienicka et al., 1981) |
| Induction of prophages in *Escherichia coli* | Not specified | S9 mix | Not specified | No induction of prophages with or without S9 mix (Szymezyk, 1981) |
| Repair test with *Salmonella typhimurium* TA 1538, TA 1978 | 50, 100 µg/ plate in DMSO | S9 mix from induced rat liver (Wistar) | Not specified | Positive without metabolic activation, ineffective with metabolic activation (Zdzienicka et al., 1981) |
| Repair test with *Salmonella typhimurium* TA 1538, TA 1978 | Not specified | Not specified | Not specified | Negative (Szymezyk, 1981) |
| *Bacillus subtilis* H17 $Rec^+$ M 45 $Rec^-$ | 2 µg/plate in DMSO | Not specified | Not specified | Positive in the Rec-Assay (Shirasu et al., 1976) |

| | | | | |
|---|---|---|---|---|
| *Bacillus subtilis* H17 Rec$^+$ M 45 Rec$^-$ | Not specified | With S9 mix | Not specified | Positive in the Rec-Assay (Kawachi et al., 1980) |
| *Escherichia coli* WP2hcr | Up to 5000 μg/plate | Not specified | Not specified | Questionable (Moriya et al., 1983) |
| *Escherichia coli* polA$^+$ and polA$^-$ | Not specified | S9 mix from Aroclor-induced rat liver | Not specified | Negative (Rosenkranz and Leifer, 1980) |
| Gene mutation in *Aspergillus nidulans* | 0, 0.5, 1, 2, 4μg/plate | S9 mix from Aroclor-induced rat liver (Wistar) | 5% reduction in survival rate at 4 μg/plate | Induction of point-mutations without metabolic activation (Zdzienicka et al., 1981) |
| Gene mutation in *Aspergillus nidulans* | Not specified | S9 mix from Aroclor-induced rat liver (Wistar) | Not specified | No induction with metabolic activation (Szymezyk, 1981) |
| *Aspergillus nidulans* | 20–40 ppm | None | Not specified | Induction of aneuploidy (Upshall and Johnson, 1981) |
| Scheduled (SDS) and unscheduled (UDS) DNA synthesis in rat thymocytes | 0.1, 1.0, 10 μg/ml | None | Not specified | Dose-dependent inhibition of DNA synthesis (SDS), no increase in unscheduled DNA-synthesis (Rocchi et al., 1980) |

**Table 2** (continued)

| Test system | Dose/ Solvent | Metabolic activation | Toxicity | Results (Reference) |
|---|---|---|---|---|
| Lung fibroblasts (hamster) | Not specified | With S9 mix | Not specified | Did not cause chromosomal aberrations (Kawachi et al., 1980) |
| SCE test in hamster ovary cells | $10^{-7}$–$10^{-5}$ M in acetone | S9 mix from Clophen-induced rat liver | Toxic from $5\times10^{-6}$ M | Negative (Donner et al., 1983) |
| SCE test in hamster ovary cells | $10^{-7}$–$10^{-5}$ M in acetone | S9 mix from Clophen-induced rat liver | Not specified | Positive (Zdzienicka et al., 1984) |
| SCE test in human lymphocytes | $10^{-7}$–$10^{-5}$ M in acetone | S9 mix from Clophen-induced rat liver | Not specified | Positive (Zdzienicka et al., 1984) |
| V 79 cells HGPRT test | 0.01–10.0 µg/ml in ethanol | None | Dose-dependent decrease in survival rate of the cells | Dose-dependent muta-genic effect (Paschin and Bakhitova, 1985) |

| | | | | |
|---|---|---|---|---|
| HGPRT test (CHO) | $10^{-7}$–5× $10^{-7}$ M | With and without S9 mix | Dose-dependent decrease in survival rate of cells | Not mutagenic (Zdzienicka et al., 1984) |
| in vivo | | | | |
| Micronucleus test male and female mice (CBA x C57B1/6J)$F_1$ | Single i.p. dose of 100 mg/kg. Bone marrow preparation 24, 36 or 48 hours after administration | – | Dose used corresponds to 25% of the $LD_{50}$ in the strain employed | Increase in the number of micronuclei at all three time points with a maximum at 24 hours (1000 polychromatic erythrocytes per mouse evaluated) (Paschin and Bakhitova, 1985) |
| Micronucleus test Chinese hamster male and female | Single dose of 0.1, 0.2 or 0.5 mg/kg in olive oil. Killed 30 hours after administration | – | Not specified | No increase in the number of micronuclei in 2000 polychromatic and 2000 normochromatic erythrocytes (Donner et al., 1983) |

**Table 2** (continued)

| Test system | Dose/ Solvent | Metabolic activation | Toxicity | Results (Reference) |
|---|---|---|---|---|
| Micronucleus test BALB/c mice, male | 2 doses of 100, 500 or 1000 mg/kg given i.p. 24 hours apart. Mice killed 6 hours after the second dose | – | 2 out of 5 mice died at 1000 mg/kg | Dose-dependent increase in the number of micro-nuclei ($p<0.001$) from 500 mg/kg (Dulout et al., 1982) |
| Micronucleus test Swiss-Webster mice | 12.5–100 mg/kg/day. 2 doses 24 hours apart | – | 200 mg/kg lethal | Dose-dependent increase in micronuclei from 50 mg/kg (Paik and Lee, 1977) |
| Micronucleus test | Oral 300–1200 mg/kg 2 doses i.p. 14–140 mg/kg | – | Not specified | Increase in micronuclei from 300 mg/kg (oral) or 18.7 mg/kg (i.p.) (Hu, 1987) |

| | | | | |
|---|---|---|---|---|
| Drosophila recessive lethal test | 1–5 mg/ml feed | – | Not specified | Significant increase in recessive lethal mutations. No dose dependency (Donner et al., 1983) |
| Silkworm | Not specified | – | Not specified | Mutagenic (Kawachi et al., 1980) |
| Rat in vivo bone marrow | Not specified | – | Not specified | Causes chromosomal aberrations (Kawachi et al., 1980) |
| Changes to mouse sperm (CFW x C57B1)$F_1$ | Single dose of 50 or 100 mg/kg, or 30 mg/kg thiram in corn oil on 5 consecutive days | – | Not specified | No effect on sperm morphology 1 week after treatment. Significant increase in morphologically-changed sperm at all three doses five weeks after treatment (Zdzienicka et al., 1982) |
| Changes to spermatocytes and sperm from Swiss albino mice | 80, 200, 320 mg/kg in acacia resin as 3 doses on 3 consecutive days | – | Highest dose is maximum sublethal dose | Dose-dependent numerical increase in abnormal sperm and aberrations in spermatocytes (Prasad et al., 1980) |

the controls. In the thiram-treated rats, a significant reduction was seen in the spontaneous incidence of leukaemias, compared with the controls, and there was a similar trend towards a reduced incidence of pituitary and thyroid tumours (Takahashi et al., 1983).

Groups of 50 male and 50 female Fischer 344 rats were given thiram in their feed at concentrations of 0, 0.05 or 0.1% for 104 weeks. In the treatment groups, the average body weight was significantly reduced, particularly in the females of the high-dose group. Feed intake was reduced in all treated animals. The survival rate was normal in males at both dose levels and in the low-dose females. Females in the high-dose group had a slightly reduced life-span. Clinical studies revealed a statistically significant increase in erythrocytes in the high-dose males, but this was not dose-dependent and was interpreted as being fortuitous. The number of white blood cells in rats without leukaemia in the thiram-treated groups was comparable to the control level for the males, but was lower in the females. This was consistent with the histopathological findings, which revealed a decreased leukaemia incidence in the thiram-treated groups. Clinical-chemical studies suggested a slight impairment of liver function in the males, although this was not associated with any histopathological changes. At post-mortem, a range of non-neoplastic changes was found in all groups, including the control group. However, no specific effects were observed that could be attributed to the thiram treatment. The incidence of neoplastic changes did not suggest a significant increase for any type of tumour in the thiram-treated groups. The reported tumour types correspond to the spontaneous tumours in Fischer rats. The other effects (reduction in body weight and blood effects) showed that the highest dose (0.1%) is very close to the maximum tolerated dose. From this the authors concluded that thiram had no carcinogenic effect, but it did reduce the incidence of spontaneous leukaemia (Hasegawa et al., 1988).

The tumour incidence was similarly not increased in the chronic feeding study discussed in Sect. 7.5 (Lee et al., 1978).

In a further carcinogenicity study, 24 male and 24 female Fischer 344 rats each received 500 ppm thiram in their feed for 122 weeks (males) or 127 weeks (females). No treatment-related tumours were observed. When the rats were also given 2000 ppm sodium nitrite in addition to thiram (500 ppm), they developed tumours of the nasal cavities (18/42 males and 15/24 females, same protocol as before).This type of tumour did not occur in the control group. Moreover, there was an increased incidence of papillomas in the fore-stomachs of the rats (Lijinsky, 1984).

In a further study (with the same strain and numbers of animals as described by Innes et al., 1969) mice received a single subcutaneous injection of 46.6 mg thiram/kg body weight (in 0.5% gelatine) at 28 days of age, and were observed up until week 78. At that time 16 out of 18 mice were still alive in 3 groups and 17 out of 18 in one group. The tumour incidence was no higher than in the control group (NTIS, 1968).

7.8 Reproductive toxicity

Eleven female albino rats were given 100 mg thiram/kg orally on day 1 and day 3 of oestrus. Males were given the same dose twice within a period of 3 days. The animals were subsequently mated. In a further group, 12 females received 100 mg thiram/kg on days 4 and 11 of pregnancy, and were mated with untreated males. On day 19 of pregnancy, the animals were killed. The number of corpora lutea and the number of live and dead foetuses were determined. No toxic effects were observed in the dams. Embryonic mortality increased from 10.9% in the controls to 24.3% in the first group (administration before pregnancy) and 26.6% in the second group (administration during pregnancy; Aleksandrov,1982).

Thiram was administered orally to female rats (5–8 animals/group, strain not specified) for 6 months at doses of 0.05, 0.1, 0.5, 1.0, 5.0 or 25.0 mg/kg (frequency of application not specified). At the end of the treatment, the females were mated with untreated males. The rats were killed on day 22 of pregnancy. The dams showed no symptoms of toxicity at doses of up to 0.5 mg/kg. Weight loss occurred at 5.0 and 25.0 mg/kg, while at 25.0 mg/kg liver damage (proliferation of the Kupffer's cells, cell lysis and pyknosis) and kidney damage (epithelial dystrophy of the tubules) were also seen. The number of resorptions increased by 25.6% and 19% at 5.0 and 25.0 mg/kg thiram respectively. No resorptions occurred in the control group (Vasilos and Anisimova, 1978).

In a further study group, females were given 25 mg thiram/kg daily throughout pregnancy. Symptoms of maternal toxicity were observed, but there was no effect on reproduction (no further details; Vasilos and Anisimova, 1978).

Following oral administration of 300 mg thiram/kg on day 4 or day 15 of pregnancy, rats exhibited apathy, loss of appetite and histological protein dystrophy of the parenchymatous organs. In the foetuses, there was an 18.4% increase in mortality compared with the controls, as well as a reduction in weight (3.3 g compared with 5.1 g in the controls). No toxic effects were seen following administration of 30 mg/kg on day 4 or day 15 of pregnancy. The authors considered the effects on reproduction to be a consequence of maternal toxicity (Vasilos and Anisimova, 1978).

Further studies on the reproductive toxicity of thiram in rats have produced the following results; inhalation of 3.8 or 0.45 mg thiram/$m^3$ for 4.5 months caused changes in the duration of oestrus (lengthening of dioestrus). The relative ovary weight increased. Female rats exposed to 1 mg thiram/$m^3$ for 4 months showed changes in the duration of oestrus. The ovaries exhibited follicular atresia. Males that were likewise exposed to 1 mg/$m^3$ for 4 months showed a decreased sperm count, degeneration of the spermatogenic epithelium and multi-nucleated giant cells. Intragastric administration of thiram to male rats at doses of 1.0 or 0.04 mg/kg for 6 months caused no damage to the gonads. Embryotoxic effects occurred after 4.5 months exposure to thiram dust (3.8 or 4.5 mg/$m^3$) by inhalation. Embryonic mortality increased, while foetal weight and the number of foetuses per dam were reduced. The threshold dose of thiram with respect to reproductive toxicity was 0.1 mg/kg (no further details; Zhavoronkov, 1979).

Female rabbits given thiram in their feed at a dose of 1% of the $LD_{50}$ (exact dose and duration of administration not specified), showed a reduction in the number of live foetuses to 60.5% of the control value on day 14 of pregnancy. The average weight of the embryos was 77.3% of that of the control animals and the average number of offspring per rabbit was 5.35 in the test group compared with 8.35 in the control group. In the treatment group, 9.4% of the offspring had deformities (type not specified) and 76% of the offspring died within 2 months. The weight of the animals that survived 4 months was 48.1% of that of the control group (no further details could be obtained from the English summary of this Russian paper). Similar findings (gonadotoxic, embryotoxic and teratogenic effects) were also seen in pigs and poultry (Zhavoronkov, 1979).

Groups of 17–20 female mice of two different strains (NMRI or SD) were given thiram (in groundnut oil) by stomach tube from day 6 to day 17 of pregnancy (12 applications) at the following doses: 5, 10, 20 or 30 mg per mouse, corresponding to 179, 357, 714 and 1071 mg/kg body weight respectively in NMRI mice and 250, 500, 1000 and 1500 mg/kg body weight respectively in SD mice. The volume administered was 0.1 ml, control animals receiving a corresponding amount of groundnut oil. The investigation was conducted in two parts; a breeding study in which mice received 5, 10 or 20 mg, 12 times post-coitum, and 3 generations of offspring of the middle-dose group were simultaneously studied; and a Caesarian study in which females of both strains were given 15, 20 or 30 mg, twice at various times during pregnancy (Roll, 1971), described as follows.

Breeding study

Administration of 10 or 20 mg/mouse produced a dose-dependent statistically significant increase ($p<0.0027$) in the rate of stillbirths (14.3 and 69.2% respectively) compared with the controls (1.4%), while a dose of 5 mg/mouse (4.3%) did not cause any difference ($p<0.14$). The number of offspring that died during the breeding period was comparable in the treatment and control groups. At 10 and 20 mg/mouse, 23.4% and 19% respectively of the animals died compared with the control (4.2%), while at 5 mg/mouse 5.8% of the offspring died. The total mortality was consequently 5.6% for the controls, 10.1% for the 5 mg group, 33.3% for the 10 mg group and 92.6% for the 20 mg group. The main cause of death was pronounced cleft palates, which were seen in one out of 139 foetuses (0.7%) in the 5 mg group, in an average of 22.3 out of 150 foetuses (15.1%) in the 10 mg group (over three generations), and in 65 out of 107 foetuses (60.8%) in the 20 mg group. At the same time, significantly lower birth weights and weights at weaning were seen at the two higher doses. Following the Caesarian section on day 18 post-coitum, the 20 mg group showed a reduced number of foetal implantations, lower foetal weight, skeletal anomalies (cleft palates, micrognathia, kyphoses) and retarded development (incomplete ossification of the calcaneus, cervical vertebral bodies and phalanges). These findings were not seen in the 10 mg group.

Treatment at specific stages of pregnancy

In order to test the sensitivity of different stages of pregnancy, NMRI mice (and also in some cases SD-mice) were treated at various times throughout pregnancy. Administration on days 6 and 7 or days 14 and 15 produced signs of embryotoxicity (increased rate of resorptions) and retarded development. Skeletal anomalies (described above) were seen following administration on days 10 and 11, and to an even greater extent on days 12 and 13 of pregnancy. The most sensitive stage with regard to organotropic malformations was the end of the embryonic phase and the beginning of the foetal development phase. In addition, there was a clear dose-response relationship in the frequency of deformities (Roll, 1971).

These findings were confirmed by Matthiaschk (1973), who also demonstrated that simultaneous intraperitoneal administration of L-cysteine reduced the total incidence and the severity of the malformations.

Robens (1969) showed that thiram (250 mg/kg body weight administered orally during organogenesis) was teratogenic in hamsters causing deformed ribs,shortened tails and umbilical hernias.

Repeatead administration of thiram to laying hens during the laying period (total 168 mg/kg body weight) caused a reduction in laying performance (up to 19%), an increase in the number of infertile eggs (49.2%), reduced rate of hatching as well as weight retardation and delayed post-embryonic development. Deformities of the extremities (11.3%, no further details) showed that thiram had teratogenic effects (Zhavoronkov and Antsiferov, 1972).

Page (1975) observed similar effects in hens given 10, 20 or 40 ppm thiram in their feed, the brood showing bilateral curvature of the toes, exophthalmus and shortened femurs.

The lack of contractility of the uterus in quails after repeated oral administration of 50 ppm thiram was associated with the laying of immature eggs with thin, soft shells. Studies on the egg-containing uteri of thiram-treated quail hens also showed a reduced ability to contract of treatment with vasopressin. This may possibly be due to an impairment of the adrenergic/cholinergic balance in the uterus (Egberts et al., 1972).

Delayed development of the testes and degeneration of the seminiferous tubule epithelia was seen in roosters on oral administration of thiram (dose not specified; Rasul and Howell, 1974).

Short (1976) reportes infertility in male rats given 132 mg thiram/kg body weight daily for about 13 weeks.

Korhonen et al. (1982) studied the embryotoxicity of thiram in hens' eggs. In this experiment, 40–50 hens' eggs (breed: white leghorn) were incubated for 3 days at 37.8 °C. Thiram in 5 μl acetone was then inroduced into the air chambers of each group of eggs at levels of 5, 10, 20, 40, 60, 80 or 100 nmol thiram/egg. The eggs were then incubated under the same conditions until day 14 (11th day after addition of the test solution). The eggs and the embryos were examined for mortality and deformities during and after the incubation period. Mortality in the embryos (to the end of day 2 of exposure) increased dose-dependently up to 88% (over-all mortality in all treated groups 48%), and further deaths occurred between days 5 and 14 of incubation (3% non-malformed, 8% malformed). 11% of the surviving birds (35 of the 332 birds used) were found to have malformations. In the embryos which died prematurely, the main malformations included changes to the eyes (lid and corneal defects) open coeloms, and deformities of the back and the neck. A similar picture was seen in the surviving birds.

Groups of 12 male and 12 female rats (age and origin not specified) were given 48 ppm thiram in their feed for 3 generations. Growth, mortality and blood composition were unaffected. Macroscopic and histological examinations revealed no treatment-related changes. Reproductive parameters (no further details) were similarly not impaired (van Esch, 1976).

7.9 Effects on the immune system

No information available.

7.10 Neurotoxicity

Behavioural studies were carried out on the offspring of female Wistar rats that had received 25 mg thiram/kg orally during pregnancy (day of treatment not specified). In the open field test, spontaneous and exploratory activity was measured on 3 consecutive days in males and females at the age of 34–36 days. The offspring of treated animals showed increased motor activity compared with the controls, independent of sex (Hinkova and Vergieva, 1976).

7.11 Other effects

In a study involving the administration of toxic doses of thiram in combination with other pesticides (such as Carbaryl, Propoxur, Pirimor, Chlorfenvinphos, Malathion, Lindane and Carbendazim), Wysocka-Paruszevska et al. (1980) showed that thiram induced both synergistic and antagonistic effects in the animals.

Fenyvesi et al. (1985) produced similar findings in combination studies with drugs that affect the central nervous system. A synergistic effect was seen in combination with Promethazine and Meprobramate. In the case of trihexylphenyl, only an additive effect was observed. In this case the evaluation was not based on equitoxic doses, but was estimated with the aid of behaviourial studies (activity, open-field test).

Short et al. (1977) showed that the toxicity of vinylidene chloride in mice could be reduced by adding thiram to the feed. This indicates a protective or antagonistic effect of thiram in vinylidene chloride poisoning. It was also established that 24 hours after thiram administration, the hepatocytes showed reductions in the enzyme complex, cytochrome P450, and in N-demethylase activity, and increased sorbitol dehydrogenase and serumglutamate transaminase activity.

Several authors have demonstrated the influence of thiram on intermediary metabolism, both in vivo and in vitro. Thus Leyck and Freundt (1981) reported an effect on fat metabolism following radioactive labelling (no further information).

Repeated oral administration of 600 ppm thiram (ca. 60 mg/kg) in the feed of male Wistar rats (weight ca. 100 g) for 15 days resulted in increased lipid levels in the liver, including total lipids, longer-chain aryl acid compounds, triglycerides and glycolipids. The glucose requirement was increased in rats under stress conditions (increased work performance, cold). The authors concluded that a disturbance of glycolysis was responsible for the accumulation of lipids in the liver (Faudemay et al. 1975).

Schreiner and Freundt (1985) demonstrated clear effects (increased activity) on epoxide hydrolase and glutathione S-transferase in the liver.

Owens (1953) showed that in vitro thiram had a marked effect on pancreatic amylase, maltase and polyphenol oxidase, although catalytic activity remained more or less unaffected.

Korablev and Simorot (1965) observed that on oral administration, respiratory enzymes (cytochrome c oxidase) were also affected (no further information).

Treatment of rats and hamsters with thiram led to inhibition of dopamine β-hydroxylase with a consequent inhibitory effect on the conversion of dopamine to noradrenaline (Lippmann and Lloyd, 1771; Maj et al., 1971).

With the aid of further in vitro studies it was established that thiram is able to form dimethylnitrosamine on incubation with nitrites (Egert and Greim, 1975).

## 8. Experience in humans

Symptoms described in man following acute contact with thiram include headaches, vomiting, heart arrhythmias, breathing difficulties, liver damage, bronchitis, decreased blood pressure, eosinophilia, lymphocytopenia and neutrocytopenia (Antonovich and Vekshtein, 1977).

Comparable effects were seen on longer contact with thiram. In addition, atrophy of the respiratory tract, inflammation of the mucous membranes of the mouth, conjunctivitis, neuritis, icterus, myocardial dystrophy, enlargement of the thyroid glands and disturbances in liver function were reported in 223 workers (42 men and 181 women, age 20–50 years) who had been employed in a seed-treatment plant for more than three years (Chepak et al., 1971).

In another cohort of 105 workers, one individual developed an adenocarcinoma of the thyroid gland and 7 others showed changes to the thyroid gland (Kaskievich and Bezugly, 1973). Measurements of exposure to nitrosamines in the rubber industry from 1979 to 1983 (25 separate measurements in 19 factories of 14 different companies) showed that dimethylnitrosamine, a contaminant in thiram, can be measured in the surrounding air at practically all stages of production. However, particularly high concentrations occur during sulphuration and vulcanization, in which thiram is used as an accelerator. Values in the breathing zones of workers were 40–90 $\mu g/m^3$ air. Values of 500–1060 $\mu g/m^3$ were measured in the air near to production processes (Spiegelhalder and Preussmann, 1983).

Yurchenko et al. (1976) reported neurosomatic changes in workers following repeated long-term contact with thiram. These changes were described as dysfunctions of cortical and brain structures, and a tendency towards hypersensitivity. Also reported was a decrease in hormonally-controlled thyroid gland function and hyperplasia of the thyroid, along with increased secretion of adrenaline and noradrenaline. The copper content and ceruloplasmin-activity of the blood were also reduced.

With regard to a sensitizing effect in humans, a number of authors give examples of cases and test results. These indicate a weak to clear allergic effect following contact with thiram, which may present as Schönlein-Henoch purpura (Sidorenko et al., 1980; Dooms-Goossens et al., 1986; Duell and Morten, 1987; van Ketel, 1984; Marks and Rainey, 1984; Rudzki and Napiorkovska, 1980; Marzulli and Maibach, 1976; Lisi et al., 1987; Weinstein and Fellner, 1979; Foussereau and Cavelier, 1977; Goitre et al., 1981; Bear and Rosenthal, 1954; Blank, 1956; Shelley, 1964; Bandmann and Naseman, 1958; Schultheiss, 1957).

Complications during pregnancy, birth and lactation occured in female workers involved in seed disinfection. Toxicosis during pregnancy and post-natal haemorrhages were observed, the incidence of which appeared to be higher in workers who came into contact with thiram, among other substances (no further details; Verzhanskii, 1976).

## 9. Threshold limit values

MAK-value since 1958, 5 $mg/m^3$ air; Pregnancy: group D (DFG,1976). 1 $mg/m^3$ air (ACGIH, 1987).

## References

ACGIH (American Conference of Governmental Industrial Hygienists)
Documentation of the threshold limit values and biological exposure indices (573.1–573.3)
5th edition, 1976 (update 1987)

Aleksandrov, S.E.
Effect of vulcanisation accelerators on embryonic mortality in rats
Bull. Exp. Biol. Med., 93, 107–109 (1982)

Andrews, A.W., Fornwald, J.A., Lijinsky, W.
Nitrosation and mutagenicity of some amine drugs
Toxicol. Appl. Pharmacol., 52, 237–244 (1980)

Antonovich, E.A., Vekshtein, M.S.
TMTD toxicolocy and the aspect of its application hygiene in agriculture
In: Pesticide application hygiene, toxicology and the clinical picture of poisonings, Kiev
VNIIGINTOX, Issue 8, 221–240 (1970)

Antonovich, E.A.
On the distribution, accumulation, metabolism and discharge of dithiocarbamates from the organism
In: Pesticide application hygiene, toxicology and the clinical picture of poisoning
M., Meditsina Publ., Issue 10, 97–105 (1973)

Antsiferov, S.D., Zhavoronkov, N.J.
Effect of TMTD on the reproductive function of animals
Veterinariya (Moscow), 2, 70–72 (1978)

Baer, R.L., Rosenthal, S.A.
The germicidal action on human skin of soap containing tetramethylthiuram disulfide
J. Invest. Dermatol., 23, 193–211 (1954)

Bandmann, H.J., Naseman, T.
Pseudopolyvalentes Kontaktekzem bei Sensibilisierung gegen das in Gummi und neuesten Arzneimitteln enthaltene Tetramethylthiuramdisulfid
Hautarzt, 9, 40 (1958)

Blank, J.H.
Allergic hypersensitivity to an antiseptic wrap
J. Am. Med. Ass., 160, 1225–1226 (1956)

Brieger, H.
Toxicity and toxicology of several accelerators used in the rubber industry
Ind. Med., 16, 473–474 (1947)

Brune, H.
Toxikologische Untersuchungen zu Thiram im chronischen Fütterungsversuch an NMRI-Mäusen
Beratungsforum für Präventivmedizin und Umweltschutz GmbH, Hamburg (1980)

Brusilovskiy, Y.S., Fiallkovskiy, A.M.
Experimental study of the skin allergic reaction of TMTD
Vestr. Dermatol. Venerol., 47, 28–31 (1973)

Chepak, V.V., Bezunglyi, V.P., Kaskevich, L.M.
Sanitary-hygienic characteristics of working conditions and health of persons working with TMTD
Vrach. Delo, 10, 136–139 (1971)

Dalvi, R.R.
Dose-dependent liver toxicity of thiram administered intraperitoneally to rats
J. Environ. Biol., 8, 25–31 (1987)

Dalvi, R.R., Deoras,D.P.
Metabolism of a dithiocarbamate fungicide thiram to carbon disulfide in the rat and its hepatotoxic implications
Acta Pharmacol. Toxicol., 58, 38–42 (1986)

Dalvi, R.R., Robbins, T.J., Williams, M.K., Deoras, D.P., Donastory, F., Banks,C.
Thiram induced toxic liver injury in male Sprague-Dawley rats
J. Environ. Sci. Health, 19, 703–712 (1984)

DFG (Deutsche Forschungsgemeinschaft)
Thiram – Toxikologisch-arbeitsmedizinische Begründung von MAK-Werten
VCH, Weinheim (1976)

Donner, M., Husgafrel-Tussiainen, K., Jenssen, D., Rannug, A.
Mutagenicity of rubber additives and curing fumes
Scand. J. Work Environ. Health, 9 (2), 27–37 (1983)

Dooms-Goossens, A.E., Debusschere, K.M., Gevers, D.M., Dupré, K.M., Degreef, H.J., Loncke, J.P., Snauwaert, J.E.
Contact dermatitis caused by airborne agents
J.Am. Acad. Dermatol., 15, 1–10(1986)

Duell, P.B., Morton, W.E.
Henoch-Schönlein purpura following thiram exposure
Arch. Intern. Med., 147, 778–779 (1987)

Dulout, F.N., Olivero, O.A., Pastori, M.C.
The mutagenic effect of thiram analysed by the micronucleus test and the anaphase-telophase test
Mutat. Res., 105, 409–412 (1982)

Egberts, J., Roos, J., Beijer, H.J.M.
Toxicity of TMTD in Japanese quail
TNO Nieuws, 27, 594–598 (1972)

Egert, G., Greim, H.
Formation of dimethylnitrosamine from pesticides carrying methylated tertiary amino-groups in the presence of nitrite and pH3
Food Cosmet. Toxicol., 14, 193–195(1976)

Esch, van G.L. (1956)
cited in: WHO (1965)

Faudemay, F., Griffaton, G., Dupuy, F., Rozen, R., Lowy, R.
Efects à court terme de pégunes à teneur élevée en dithiocarbamates sur le métabolisme glucidique et lipique du foie de rat
Am. Nutr. Alim., 29, 371–394 (1975)

Fenyvesi, G., Botos, M., Ivan, J.
Pesticide-drug interaction in rats
Arch. Toxicol., 8, 269–271 (1985)

Foussereau, J., Cavelier, C.
La N-isopropyl-N'-phénylparaphénylénediamine a-t-elle sa place dans la batterie standard d'allergèns? Importance de cet allergène dans l'intolerance au caoutchouc
Dermatologica, 155, 164–167 (1977)

Freundt, K.J., Netz, H.
Behaviour of blood acetaldehyde in alcohol-treated rats following administration of Thirams
Drug Research, 27, 105–108 (1977)

Goitre, M., Bedello, P.G., Cane, D.
Allergic dermatitis and oral challenge to tetramethylthiuram disulfide
Contact Dermatitis, 7, 272–273 (1981)

Griepentrog, F.
Allergiestudien mit einfachen chemischen Substanzen
5. Mitteilung: Thiurame
Arzneimittel-Forsch., 10, 542–544 (1960)

Griepentrog, F.
Cerebrale Pseudokalkablagerungen bei chronischer Intoxikation mit Thiuramen im Tierversuch
Archiv für Psychiatrie und Zeitschrift f. d. ges. Neurologie, 202, 412–422 (1961)

Griepentrog, F.
Tumorartige Schilddrüsenveränderungen in chronisch-toxikologischen Tierversuchen mit Thiuramen
Beitr. Path. Arch., 126, 243–255 (1962)

Hasegawa, R., Takehashi, M., Furukawa, F., Tryoda, K., Sato, H., Jang, J.J., Hayashi, Y.
Carcinogenicity study of thiram in F 344 rats
Toxicology, 51, 155–165 (1988)

Hedenstedt, A., Rannug, U., Ramel, C., Wachtmeister, C.A.
Mutagenicity and metabolism studies on 12 thiuram and dithiocarbamate compounds used as accelerators in the Swedish rubber industry
Mutat. Res., 68, 313–325 (1979)

Hinkova, L., Vergieva, T.
Behaviourial studies on the progeny of pesticide-treated rats during pregnancy
Adverse effects of Environmental Chemicals and Psychotropic Drugs, 2, 215–218 (1976)

Hu, Y., Wang, N., Kong, C., You, X.
Application of micronucleus test for detection of cytogenic effects of tetramethylthiuramdisulfide
Huanjing Kexue, 8, 30–32 (1987)

Innes, J.R.M., Ulland, B.M., Valerio, M.G., Petrucelli, L., Fishbein, L., Hart, E.R., Pallote, A.J., Bates, R.R., Falke, H.L., Gart, J.J., Klein, M., Mitchell, J., Peters, J.
Bioassay of pesticides and industrial chemicals for tumorigenicity in mice: a preliminary note
J. Natl. Cancer Inst., 42, 1101–1114 (1969)

IPS (Industrieverband Pflanzenschutz e.V.)
Wirkstoffe in Pflanzenschutz- und Schädlingsbekämpfungsmitteln (1982)

Izmerov, N.F. (ed.)
Scientific reviews of Soviet literature on toxicity and hazards of chemicals; 12, Thiram
United Nations Environment Programme (UNEP) International Register of Potentially Toxic Chemicals (IRPTC) (1982)

Kaskievich, L.M., Bezugly, V.P.
Clinical aspects of intoxications induced by TMTD
Vrach. Delo, 6, 128–130 (1973)

Kawachi, T., Komatsu, I., Kada, T., Ishidate, M., Sasaki, M., Sugiyama, T., Tazima, Y.
Results of recent studies on the relevance of various shortterm screening tests in Japan
Applied Methods in Oncology, 3, 253–267 (1980)

Khoroshilova, N.V., Salnikova, L.S., Domshlatz, M.G., Chirkova, E.M.
Mutagenic and gonadotropic activities of thiuram EF
Gig. Tr. Prof. Zabol., 3, 20–22 (1980)

Korablev, M.V., Simorot, R.P.
The influence exerted by dithiocarbaminic acid derivates on the enzymatic activity of cytochromoxidase, succinodehydrogenase and catalase
Farmakol. Toksikol., 28, 234–237 (1965)

Korhonen, A., Hemminki, K., Vainio, H.
Application of the chicken embryo in testing for embryotoxicity, Thiurams
Scand. J. Work Environ. Health, 8, 63–69 (1982)

Kurata, Y., Furukawa, F., Kokulo, T.
Oral subchronic toxicity test for tetramethylthiuramdisulfide in F344 Du Crj rat
Eisei Shikenjo Hokoku, 98, 69–76 (1980)

Lee, C.C., Russel, J.Q., Minor, J.L.
Oral toxicity of ferbam and thiram in rodents
J. Toxicol. Environ. Health, 4, 93–106 (1978)

Leyck, S., Freundt, K.J.
Thiram-induced disturbance of microsomal phospholipid bioformation and phospholipid fatty acid pattern
J. Toxicol. Environ. Health, 7, 533–545 (1981)

Lijinsky, W.
Induction of tumors of the nasal cavity in rats by concurrent feeding of Thiram and sodium nitrite
J. Toxicol. Environ. Health, 13, 609–614 (1984)

Lippmann, W., Lloyd, K.
Effects of tetramethylthiuramdisulfide and structurally-related compounds on the dopamine-β-hydroxylase activity in the rat and hamster
Arch. Int. Pharmacodyn. Ther., 189, 348–357 (1971)

Lisi, P., Caraffini, S., Assalve, D.
Irritation and sensitization potential of pesticides
Contact Dermatitis, 17, 212–218 (1987)

Lowy, R., Griffaton, G., Dupuy, F., Ardouin, B., Manchon, P.
Dietary no-effect level of a dithiocarbamate fungicide, thiram, evaluated from measurement data on rats
J. Toxicol. Environ. Health, 6, 403–419 (1980)

Maj, J., Sowinska, J., Baran, L.
Central action of ethyldimethyldithiocarbamate and analogous carbamate derivatives
Diss. Pharm. Pharmacol., 23, 25–31 (1971)

Marks, J.G., Rainey, M.A.
Cutaneous reactions to surgical preparations and dressings
Contact Dermatitis, 10, 1–5 (1984)

Marzulli, F.N., Maibach, H.J.
Contact allergy: Predictive testing in man
Contact Dermatitis, 2, 1–17 (1976)

Matthiaschk, G.
Über den Einfluß von L-Cystein auf die Teratogenese durch Thiram (TMTD) bei NMRI-Mäusen
Arch. Toxicol., 30, 251–262 (1973)

Moriya, M., Kato, K., Shirasu, Y., Koda, T.
Mutagenicity screening of pesticides in microbial systems
Mutat. Res., 54, 221 (1978)

Moriya, M., Oate, T., Watanabe, K., Miyazawa, T., Kato, K., Shirasu, Y.
Further mutagenicity studies on pesticides in bacterial reversion assay system
Mutat. Res., 116, 185–216 (1983)

NTIS (National Technical Information Service)
Evaluation of carcinogenic, teratogenic and mutagenic activities of selected pesticides and industrial chemicals, Vol. 1
U.S. Department of Commerce, Washington DC (1968)

Owens, R.G.
Studies on the nature of fungicidal action
Boyse Thompson, 17, 221–243 (1953)

Page, R.K.
Teratogenic activity of Arosan fed to broilers and hens
Avian Dis., 19, 463–472 (1975)

Paik, S.G., Lee, S.Y.
Genetic effects of pesticides in the mammalian cells
1. Induction of micronucleus
Korean Journal of Zoology, 20, 19–28 (1977)

Paschin, Y.V., Bakhitova, L.M.
Mutagenic effects of thiram in mammalian somatic cells
Food. Chem. Toxicol., 23, 373–375 (1985)

Prasad, M.H., Pushpavath, K., Rita, P., Reddy, P.P.
The effect of thiram on the germ cells of male mice
Food Chem. Toxicol., 25, 709–711 (1987)

Rannug, A., Rannug, U.
Enzyme inhibition as a possible mechanism of the mutagenicity of dithiocarbamine acid derivatives in *Salmonella typhimurium*
Chem. Biol. Interact., 49, 329–340 (1984)

Rannug, A., Rannug, U., Ramel, C.
Genotoxic effects of additives in synthetic elastics with special considerations to the mechanism of action of thiurams and dithiocarbamates
Prog. Clin. Biol. Res., 141, 407–419 (1984)

Rasul, A.R., Howell, J.M.
The toxicity of some dithiocarbamate compounds in young and adult domestic fowls
Toxicol. Appl. Pharmacol., 30, 63–78 (1974)

Robbins, R.C., Katelic, J.
Fate of tetramethylthiuramdisulfide in the digestive tract of the ruminant animal
J.Agric. Food. Chem., 9, 256–260 (1961)

Robens, J.F.
Teratologic studies of carbaryl, diazon, urea, disulfiram and thiram in small laboratory animals
Toxicol. Appl. Pharmacol., 15, 152–163 (1969)

Rocchi, P., Perocev, P., Alberghini, W., Fini, A., Prodi, G.
Effect of pesticides on scheduled and unscheduled DNA-synthesis of rat thymocytes and human lymphocytes
Arch. Toxicol., 45, 101–108 (1980)

Roll, R.
Teratologische Untersuchungen mit Thiram an zwei Mäusestämmen
Arch. Toxikol., 27, 173–186 (1971)

Rosenkranz, H., Leifer, Z.
Determining the DNA modifying activity of chemical using DNA-polymerase-deficient *Escherichia coli*
Chem. Mutagens, 6, 109–147 (1980)

Rudzki, E., Napiorkovska, T.
Dermatitis caused by the Polish fungicide Sadoplon 75
Contact Dermatitis, 6, 300–301 (1980)

Schreiner, E., Freundt, K.J.
Activities of hepatic epoxide hydrolase and glutathione α-transferase in rats under the influence of tetramethylthiuramdisulfide, tetramethylthiurammonosulfide and dimethyldithiocarbamate
Toxicol. Lett., 25, 147–152 (1985)

Schultheiss, E.
Zur therapeutischen Anwendung von Tetramethylthiuramdisulfid
Derm. Wochenschr., 135, 160–162 (1957)

Shelley, W.B.
Golf-course dermatitis due to thiram fungicide
J. Am. Med. Ass., 188, 415–417 (1964)

Shirasu, Y., Moriya, M., Kato, K., Furuhashi, A., Kada, T.
Mutagenic screening of pesticides in the microbial system
Mutat. Res., 40, 19–30 (1986)

Short, R.D., Russel, J.Q., Minor, J.L., Lee, C.C.
Developmental toxicity of ferric dimethyldithiocarbamate and bis(dimethylthiocarbamoyl)disulfide in rats and mice
Toxicol. Appl. Pharmacol., 35, 83–94 (1976)

Short, R.D., Winston, J.M., Minor, J.L., Hong, C.B., Seifter, J., Lee, C.C.
Toxicity of vinylidenechloride in mice and rats and its alteration by various treatments
J. Toxicol. Environ. Health, 3, 913–921 (1977)

Sidorenko, E.N., Buslenko, A.J., Bajda, N.A., Kozinceva, P.V., Ivanova, S.J., Dijacenko, E.J., Muchtarova, N.D., Titenkov, J.K.
Allergische Erkrankungen bei Arbeitern in der Gummiproduktion (German translation)
Vrach. Delo, 12, 14–16 (1980)

Spiegelhalder, B., Preussmann, R.
Occupational nitrosamine exposure. 1. Rubber and tyre industry
Carcinogenesis, 4, 1147–1152 (1983)

Stefan, A., Ceausescu, S., Stancioiu, N. (1972)
cited in: DFG (1976)

Szymezyk, T.
The mutagenicity of the fungicide thiram
Mutat. Res., 85, 223–224 (1981)

Takahashi, M., Kokubo, T., Furukawa, F., Nagano, K., Mackawa, A., Kurokawa, Y., Hayashi, Y.
Inhibition of spontaneous leukemia in F-344 rats by tetramethylthiuram disulfide (thiram)
Gann, 74, 810–813 (1983)

Upshall, A., Johnson, P.E.
Thiram-induced abnormal chromosome segregation in *Aspergillus nidulans*
Mutat. Res., 89, 297–301 (1981)

van Ketel, W.G.
Contact urticaria from rubber gloves after dermatitis from thiuram
Contact Dermatitis,11, 323–324 (1984)

Vasilos, A.E., Anisimova, L.A.
Reproduktive Funktion von Ratten bei akuter und chronischer Intoxikation mit Tetramethylthiuramdisulfid (translation from Russian)
Gig. Sanit., 6, 37–40 (1978)

Veltmann, J.R., Linton, S.S.
Influence of dietary tetramethylthiuramdisulfide on growth and incidence of tibial dyschondroplasia in single comb white leghorn chicks
Poultry Science, 65, 1205–1207 (1986)

Verzhanskii, P.S.
Effect of pesticides on the reproductive function
Khar'k. Med. Inst. Kharkov, 124, 29–32 (1976)

Vorob'eva, R.S., Kasparov, A.A.
Thiurams, tetramethyl thiuram
M. Meditsina Publ., 93–101 (1968)

Vorob'eva, R.S., Mezentseva, N.V.
Experimental study of comparative toxicity of new rubber accelerators
Gig. Tr. Prof. Zabol., 7, 28–33 (1962)

Waibl, P.E., Johnson, E.L., Pomeroy, B.S., Howard, L.B.
Toxicity of tetramethylthiuram
Science, 36, 679–703 (1957)

Weast, R.C. (ed.)
CRC-Handbook of Chemistry and Physics
62nd ed., C-270
CRC Press, Boca Raton, Florida (1981/82)

Weinstein, L.H., Fellner, M.J.
Rubber band dermatitis
Int. J. Dermatol., 18, 558 (1979)

WHO (World Health Organisation)
Evaluation of the toxicity of pesticide residues in food
WHO Food Add., 27, 181–184 (1965)

Windholz, M. (ed.)
The Merck Index
10th ed., p. 1343
Merck & Co., Rahway, USA (1983)

Worthing, C.R., Walker, S.B.
The Pesticide Manual – a world compendium
The British Crop Protection Council, 2nd ed. (1983)

Wysocka-Paruszevska, B., Osicka, A., Brzezinski, J., Gradowska, J.
An evaluation of the toxicity of thiuram in combination with other pesticides
Arch. Toxicol., 4, 449–451 (1980)

Yurchenko, J.V., Kazakevich, R.L., Sasiowich, L.M.
Neuro-somatic disorders due to prolonged effect of tetramethylthiuramdisulfide
Vrach. Delo, 4, 135–138 (1976)

Zdzienicka, M., Zielenska, M., Tudek, B., Szymczyk, T.
Mutagenic activity of thiram in Ames tester strains of *Salmonella typhimurium*
Mutat. Res., 68, 9–13 (1979)

Zdzienicka, M., Zielenska, M., Trojanowska, M., Szymczyk, T., Bignami, M., Carere, A.
Microbial short-term assays with thiram in vitro
Mutat. Res., 89, 1–7 (1981)

Zdzienicka, M., Hrymiewicz, M., Pienkowska, M.
Thiram-induced sperm-head abnormalities in mice
Mutat. Res., 102, 261–264 (1982)

Zhavoronkov, N.I.
Assessment of the effect of pesticides on reproductive function of animals
Veterinariya, 9, 67–69 (1979)

Zhavoronkov, N.I., Antsiferov, S.D.
Effects of tetramethylthiuramdisulfide on chickens
Veterinariya, 8, 92–93 (1972)

Zhilenko,V.N.
Study of the TMTD toxicity with its simultaneous entrance with water and air into the organism of rats
Gig. Tr. Prof. Zabol., 2, 42–44 (1976)

# Methoxyacetic acid

## 1. Summary and assessment

The available data show methoxyacetic acid to be of moderate acute toxicity to animals after oral administration ($LD_{50}$ rat oral, between 1000 and 1470 mg/kg body weight).

On single and repeated administration, methoxyacetic acid produces testicular atrophy. Because of this, the no-effect level for the rat on single oral administration is less than 118 mg/kg body weight, and on repeated oral dosing (for 8 days) is between 30 and 100 mg/kg body weight/day. Repeated oral doses of 100 and 300 mg/kg in rats also leads to a reduction in the thymus weight and in the number of thymocytes. The no-observed-effect level for this lies between 30 and 100 mg/kg body weight.

Undiluted methoxyacetic acid is highly corrosive to the skin of animals.

In the Salmonella/microsome test, methoxyacetic acid is not mutagenic.

Methoxyacetic acid produces malformations in the foetus. After intraperitoneal administration on days 10 or 12 of pregnancy, the no-effect level for the rat foetus is below 9 mg/kg body weight. After oral administration of 376 or 188 mg/kg body weight on day 12, malformations of the heart and extremities are seen in the rat foetuses. Methoxyacetic acid reduces the fertility of the parental and $F_1$-generation. The no-effect level for oral administration is less than 140 mg/kg body weight/day.

In addition to methoxyacetaldehyde and/or further metabolites, methoxyacetic acid is the major metabolite of methoxyethanol (ethylene glycol monomethyl ether). It has been suggested that this metabolite could be the causal factor in the teratogenicity of methoxyethanol.

The results of further studies are not available, so a complete toxicological evaluation is not possible at present. The critical factors for methoxyacetic acid seem to be its damaging effects on the testes and its embryotoxic potential.

On behalf of BG-Chemie further investigations are planned to examine the acute and sub-chronic inhalation toxicity.

## 2. Name of substance

| | | |
|---|---|---|
| 2.1 | Usual name | Methoxyacetic acid |
| 2.2 | IUPAC-name | Methoxyacetic acid |
| 2.3 | CAS-No. | 625-45-6 |

## 3. Synonyms, common and trade names

MAA
2-Methoxyacetic acid
Methoxyessigsäure

## 4. Structural and molecular formulae

4.1 Structural formula

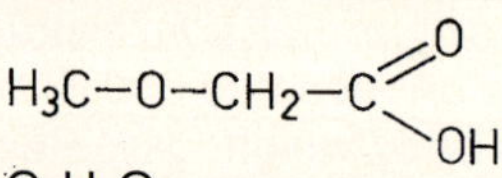

4.2 Molecular formula $C_3H_6O_3$

## 5. Physical and chemical properties

| | | |
|---|---|---|
| 5.1 | Molecular weight, g/mol | 90.09 |
| 5.2 | Melting point, °C | 7 (BASF, 1986) |
| 5.3 | Boiling point, °C | 202 (BASF, 1986) |
| 5.4 | Vapour pressure, hPa | 1.8 (at 20 °C) (BASF, 1986)<br>4.8 (at 50 °C) (BASF, 1986) |
| 5.5 | Density, $g/cm^3$ | 1.18 (at 20 °C) (BASF, 1986) |
| 5.6 | Solubility in water | Miscible in all proportions (BASF, 1986) |
| 5.7 | Solubility in organic solvents | No information available |
| 5.8 | Solubility in fat | No information available |
| 5.9 | pH-value | 1.6 (10% in water, at 20 °C) (BASF, 1986) |
| 5.10 | Conversion factor | 1 ppm $\hat{=}$ 3.74 $mg/m^3$<br>1 $mg/m^3$ $\hat{=}$ 0.27 ppm<br>(at 25 °C and 1013 hPa) |

## 6. Uses

Industrial intermediate.

## 7. Results of experiments

7.1 Toxicokinetics and metabolism

No information available

7.2 Acute and subacute toxicity

The following $LD_{50}$ values have been reported after single intraperitoneal and oral administration to 5 animals of both sexes: Mouse, i. p. between 50 and 200 mg/kg body weight; rat, oral between 1000 and 1470 mg/kg body weight. During the 14-day observation period the following symptoms of toxicity were prominent in rats and mice after oral and intraperitoneal administration: dyspnoea, apathy, abnormal position, reeling, atonia, tonic spasms, ruffled fur, cyanosis and paresis. In rats, the following macroscopic findings were seen in those that died during the experiment:

| | |
|---|---|
| Heart | acute dilation, acute congestive hyperaemia |
| Lungs | acute swelling of moderate severity |
| Stomach | extensive bloody ulceration, haemorrhagic corrosive gastritis |
| Intestine | necrosis of the mucosa, bloody contents, severe congestion of the vessels |

No macroscopic effects were seen in the rats killed at the end of the 14-day observation period. In the mice, no treatment-related macroscopic effects were found either in the animals that died during the study, or those that were killed at the end of the 14-day observation period (BASF, 1981).

The inhalation toxicity of methoxyacetic acid was studied in the inhalation risk test. This involved passing 200 l air/hour through a 5 cm-deep layer of methoxyacetic acid at 20 °C. Twelve rats were exposed to this mixture for 7 hours. Observed symptoms of toxicity included closing of the eyes, „snout wiping“ and rhinitis. No deaths occurred either during exposure or during the 14-day observation period. Autopsy revealed no macroscopic effects (BASF, 1981).

Doses of 30, 100 or 300 mg/kg body weight/day were given by stomach tube to male Fischer rats (five animals/group). The methoxyacetic acid was administered on 5 days/week for 8 days. From 100 mg/kg, there was a significant dose-dependent reduction in the absolute and relative thymus weight, the erythrocyte count, and the haemoglobin and haematocrit level ($p \leq 0.05$ in each case). In the high dose group from the 5th day of administration there were significant reductions in body weight, absolute and relative spleen and testes weights, and leucocyte count ($p \leq 0.05$ in each case). The following effects were seen from 100 mg/kg body weight, on histological examination: loss of thymocytes in the thymic cortex and atrophy of the germ cells in the seminiferous tubules („degeneration of testicular germinal epithelium"). The high dose led to reduced cell density in the bone marrow and giant cell formation in the testes. Granulopoiesis, erythropoiesis and thrombopoiesis were not affected. The spleen was not examined in this study (Miller et al., 1982).

## 7.3 Skin and mucous membrane effects

A cotton patch (ca. 2.5×2.5 cm) loaded with ca. 0.5 ml methoxyacetic acid was applied occlusively to the clipped dorsal skin of white rabbits (two or four animals/group) for 3 minutes or for 1 or 4 hours. After treatment, the application site was washed first with polyethylene glycol 400, and then with a 50% aqueous polyethylene glycol 400 solution. Evaluation of the exposed skin took place 15–30 minutes after removal of the test patch, and at 24 hours, 48 hours and 8 days after application. After a 3-minute exposure, a slight to intense reddening and marked oedema were observed in two out of four animals 24 hours after application. In the other two animals, only „questionable reddening" was reported. Three of the four animals (which were also exposed for 1 hour simultaneously) had to be killed after 2 days due to the corrosive effect. In the surviving rabbit which, after 24 hours, showed only questionable reddening, the irritant effect cleared up completely after 48 hours. Exposures of 1 or 4 hours caused a severe to very severe reddening of the skin with oedema formation, depending on the duration of exposure. In addition, moist and blistering necroses were visible. After a 1-hour exposure, three of the four animals had to be killed because of the corrosive effect, and after a 4-hour exposure both animals had to be killed. In the sole surviving animal, inflammation was still present after 8 days of observation, the skin still showing very marked reddening and slight oedema formation at that time (BASF, 1981).

The irritant effect on the eyes was not tested because of the severe corrosive effect on the skin (BASF, 1981).

## 7.4 Sensitization

No information available.

## 7.5 Subchronic and chronic toxicity

No information available.

## 7.6 Genotoxicity

### 7.6.1 In vitro

Methoxyacetic acid was tested in prokaryotes (*Salmonella typhimurium* TA 98, TA 100, TA 1535, TA 1537 and TA 1538), both with and without the addition of Aroclor 1254-induced rat liver. There were no indications of mutagenic activity (no further information given on experimental protocol or test concentrations; McGregor et al., 1983).

### 7.6.2 In vivo

No information available.

## 7.7 Carcinogenicity

No information available.

## 7.8 Reproductive toxicity

A single oral or intraperitoneal dose of 592 mg methoxyacetic acid/kg body weight given to male rats (five animals/group) caused degenerative changes (pyknosis, condensing of the cell nuclei) and loss of spermatocytes at the pachytene stage, three days after administration. There were no effects on the spermatocytes at the leptotene or zygotene stages, or on the spermatogonia or Sertoli cells. The weight of the testes was significantly reduced ($p \leq 0.001$ and $p \leq 0.01$, for oral and intraperitoneal administration, respectively). Histological examination of the epididymides, seminal vesicles, prostate and liver revealed no effects (Foster et al., 1986).

These results were confirmed in an extended study. Methoxyacetic acid was administered to male rats by stomach tube at doses of 118, 296 or 592 mg/kg body weight. Six animals/group, including a control group, were killed after 1, 2, 4 and 14 days and the testes, epididymides, seminal vesicles, prostate and liver were histopathologically examined. Reduced body weight was reported (no further details) at all doses during the first two days after administration, but this returned to normal during the observation period. The relative testis weight was significantly reduced ($p \leq 0.05$) in the high dose group from the 4th day of the experiment. In all the treated groups, dose-dependent effects were seen in the testes 24 hours after administration. In the animals of the lowest dose group, minimal damage (pyknosis, condensing of the cell nuclei) occurred in the spermatocytes at the early pachytene or diplotene stages, as well as damage to the secondary spermatocytes. After 14 days, mature spermatids were also affected. The high dose led to degenerative changes and loss of secondary spermatocytes, spermatids and spermatocytes in the zygotene, pachytene, diplotene and diakinesis stages. An increase in the number of spermatocytes at the pachytene stage was observed 14 days after exposure. An increased number of immature and abnormal cells was found in the epididymides (no further details). No effects were found in the seminal vesicles, prostate or liver on histological examination (Foster et al., 1987).

Methoxyacetic acid was administered to male Sprague-Dawley rats for 4 days by stomach tube at a dose of 592 mg/kg body weight/day. Six rats were used per dose. Methoxyacetic acid led to a significant ($p \leq 0.01$) reduction in relative testis, liver and body weights. Relative prostate and seminal vesicle weights remained unaffected. Histological examination of the testes revealed degenerative changes (pyknosis, condensing of the cell nuclei, eosinophilic cytoplasm), loss of spermatocytes at the pachytene, diplotene or diakinesis stages, and loss of secondary spermatocytes and early spermatids. There were no effects on the spermatocytes at the leptotene and zygotene stages, or on the spermatogonia or Sertoli cells. No changes were evident in the liver and epididymides. The seminal vesicles and prostate were not histologically examined (Foster et al., 1983, 1984; Gray et al., 1985).

In an embryotoxicity study, Wistar rats received 0.160 or 0.320 ml methoxyacetic acid/kg body weight orally on day 12 of pregnancy ($\hat{=}$188 or 376 mg/kg body weight). Eight animals per group and a control group (n = 13) were used. On day 20 of pregnancy, both treated groups showed an increased post-implantation loss (control 4.4%; 0.160 ml/kg 15.1%; 0.320 ml/kg 53.8%) and an increased number of foetuses with malformations (control 0.0%; 0.160 ml/kg 53.1%; 0.320 ml/kg 98.9%). The main malformations seen were hydronephrosis, malformation of the heart (perforation of the interventricular septum, levocardia, and extension of the ductus arteriosus and arcus aortae), deformities of the extremities (shortened or curved, ventral polydactylia) and shortened and bent tails. The relationship to maternally-toxic doses was not described (Scott et al., 1986; Ritter et al., 1985).

In a further teratogenicity study in Wistar-Porton rats, 2.5 mmol methoxyacetic acid/kg body weight ($\hat{=}$225 mg/kg body weight) was administered intraperitoneally to groups of eight to ten females on days 8, 10, 12 or 14 of pregnancy. The laparotomy took place on day 20 of pregnancy. Methoxyacetic acid led to increased foetal mortality which was most marked after administration on day 8 of pregnancy

(93%, control 0%). The mortality was 61% after administration on day 10 of pregnancy, 16% on day 12 of pregnancy and 3% on day 14 of pregnancy. The foetal body weight was significantly reduced in all treated groups. Methoxyacetic acid led to malformations at all treatment times, the highest rate being found on day 12 of pregnancy with 92.5% of all foetuses affected (average value per litter, control 15.4%). The main malformations seen were skeletal (fused ribs, absence of vertebrae, missing or shortened ulna, fibula and radius), hydrocephalus and urogenital malformations. The incidence of skeletal variation (incomplete ossification of skull, sternebrae and vertebrae) was highest after administration on day 8 of pregnancy at 60.0% (control 33.8%; Brown et al., 1984).

In a separate series of experiments to examine the relationship between dose and effect, groups of five pregnant rats received 0.1, 0.5, 1.0, 1.5, 2.0 or 2.5 mmol/kg i. p. on days 10 or 12 of pregnancy. The parameters assessed were foetal deaths and resorptions, and abnormal surviving foetuses including those with delayed ossification, skeletal malformations and hydrocephalus. The dams were killed on day 20. The most sensitive parameters were skeletal malformations and hydrocephalus, the incidences of which were increased over the entire dose range from 0.1 to 2.5 mmol/kg (corresponding to 9–225 mg/kg). The relationship to the maternally-toxic dose range was not described (Brown et al., 1984).

In a two-generation study on fertility and breeding, concentrations of 0.1, 0.2 or 0.4% methoxyacetic acid were administered to CD-1 mice in their drinking water. These levels correspond to doses of about 140, 240 or 390 mg methoxyacetic acid/kg body weight/day. Per dose and sex, 20 animals were used in the $F_0$-generation and 40 in the control group. The experimental design consisted of three Sections (I–III) and is further described in Fig.1. Males and females were pretreated for 7 days. The pretreatment was followed by a fertility study lasting 98 days (throughout which time the chemical was administered continuously). During this period one male and one female were kept in each cage. The young born during the 98-day breeding study were killed immediately after birth (day 0 of life). Weight, number and sex of the offspring were determined (Section I). The 98-day breeding study followed a 21-day period of isolation, both for males and females, with continuous administration of the chemical. The animals born during this period served as the $F_1$-generation in Section III. The sex-specific influence on fertility of the parents in the high-dose group was investigated after 126 days

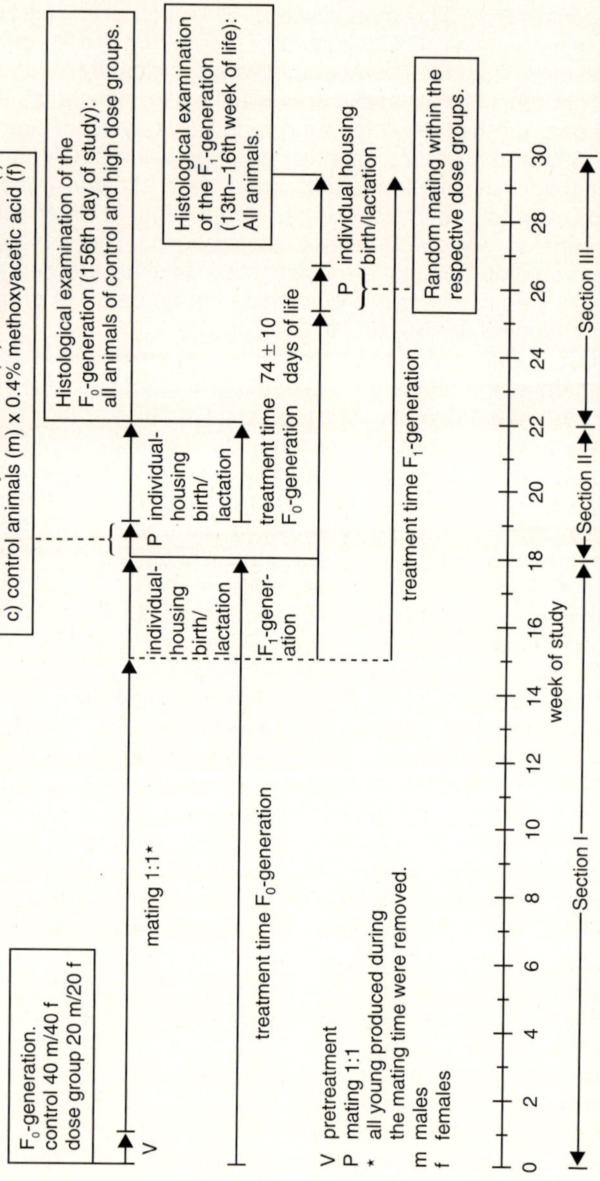


**Figure 1.** Two-generation study on reproduction and fertility assessment in CD-1 mice on oral administration of methoxyacetic acid in the drinking water (NTP, 1986)

of administration. After conclusion of the study, the parents of the control- and the high-dose groups were dissected on the 156th day of the investigation and histologically examined (liver, kidneys, adrenal glands, testes, epididymides, prostates, seminal vesicles, ovaries with fallopian tubes, uterus and vagina; Section II). A second breeding study – with continuous administration of the chemical – was carried out in the offspring of the $F_1$-generation on day 74 ± 10 of life. The doses used corresponded to those given to the parents. The animals of the $F_1$-generation were dissected in the 13th–16th week of life and histologically examined (liver, kidneys, adrenal glands, testes, epididymides, prostates, seminal vesicles, ovaries and fallopian tubes, uterus and vagina; Section III).

Results of Section I:

Concentrations of methoxyacetic acid of 0.1% and above led to both, a dose-dependent decrease in water intake in the dams (control 6.9 ml; 0.1% 5.6 ml; 0.2% 4.8 ml and 0.4% 3.9 ml/day per animal) and a reduction in body weight (18th week of study: control 50.1 g; 0.1% 40.8 g; 0.2% 37.9 g and 0.4% 33.9 g). At the high dose, vaginal bleeding occurred in four mice; these and one other dam died during the first 4 weeks of the study. One animal from the control group and one from the middle dose group also died (cause of death not specified). The fertility index[1] was 100% in the control and low-dose groups, and 95% at the middle dose. No animals were pregnant in the high dose group. The number of litters per dam, the number of live offspring per litter, the absolute body wight of surviving male offspring and the number of surviving offspring per litter, correlated with the body weight of male and female offspring were significantly reduced ($p \leq 0.1$ or $p \leq 0.05$) at 0.1% and above. The ratio of male to female offspring and the absolute body weight of the surviving female offspring was not affected. The body weight of the offspring in the low-dose group (0.1%) was significantly decreased ($p \leq 0.01$) on the 4th and 74th day after birth. Mortality in the low-dose group from day 0 to day 21 of lactation was 75.4% (control 10.3%), and from day 21 to 74 ± 10 of life was 3.2% (control 2.8%). At the middle dose (0.2%), all offspring died before the 4th day of life (no animals were pregnant in the high dose group, see above).

[1]
$$\text{fertility index} = \frac{\text{number of pregnant females}}{\text{number of treated females}} \times 100$$

Results of Section II:

On the 127th day of the study (immediately after the 21-day isolation period – see figure 1) the parents ($F_0$-generation) were again mated according to the following arrangement:

a) male control × female control.
b) treated male (0.4% methoxyacetic acid) × female control.
c) male control × treated female (0.4% methoxyacetic acid).

Sixteen to twenty pairs were used per study group. Pairing was for 7 days, during which time no administration of methoxyacetic acid took place. After the 7-day mating period, methoxyacetic acid treatment was continued up to the 155th day of the study (the same doses were used as at the beginning of the study).

The mating index [2] remained unchanged in all three study groups and was between 70% and 94%. The fertility index was 70% for study group a), 5% for group b) and 6% for group c). In group a), all pregnant dams gave birth, while in group b), only one animal became pregnant and produced four offspring. In group c), the only pregnant mouse produced no offspring. Because of the low number of offspring in the treated groups, these results could not be comparatively evaluated. Autopsy of the parents ($F_0$-generation) after the 155th day of the study revealed significantly reduced ($p \leq 0.01$) body weights, absolute and relative weights of the testes, epididymides and seminal vesicles and a significantly reduced ($p \leq 0.05$) absolute prostate weight in males of the highest dose group (0.4%). Liver, kidney and adrenal gland weights remained unaffected. Sperm motility and sperm count were reduced in the highest dose group ($p \leq 0.01$) and the number of abnormal sperm was significantly increased ($p \leq 0.01$). The absolute body weight and the absolute liver weight were significantly decreased ($p \leq 0.01$) in females at the highest dose. Absolute and relative kidney and adrenal gland weights were not affected. No pathological changes were found in the liver, kidneys, adrenal glands, prostate, ovaries, fallopian tubes, uterus or vagina, on histological examination of the animals in the highest dose group. The oestrus cycle was also unaffected. In the testes, atrophy of the seminiferous tubules and inhibition of spermatogenesis were evident. The Sertoli cells were unaffected, but the interstitial cells were hyperplastic. The number of mature sperm in the epididymides was reduced. Animals in the low- and medium-

[2]
$$\text{Mating index} = \frac{\text{number of females mated}}{\text{number of females used}} \times 100$$

dose groups were not subjected to anatomical-pathological examination.

Results of Section III:

On day 74±10 of life, the animals of the $F_1$-generation were randomly paired for 7 days within their respective dose groups (see figure 1). Administration of methoxyacetic acid (which was the same as in the parents) was continued until sacrifice (13th to 16th week of life). The control group contained 20 pairs, the 0.1% dose group 15 pairs. Further animals were not available (see above). A methoxyacetic acid concentration of 0.1% in the drinking water corresponded to a dose of 144.8 mg/kg body weight/day in the males, and 172.6 mg/kg body weight/day in the females. No mating took place between the animals of the low-dose group (0.1%). The mating and fertility indices for the control group were both 90%. On the 21st day after mating (13th–16th week of life) all the animals of the $F_1$-generation were killed and histologically examined (only animals of the low-dose group were available). In the treated males, body weight and absolute and relative testis and epididymis weights were significantly reduced ($p \le 0.01$ or $p \le 0.05$), while the relative liver weight was significantly increased ($p \le 0.01$). There were no effects on the absolute and relative weights of the kidneys, adrenal glands, prostates, seminal vesicles, or on the absolute liver weight. Sperm motility and the sperm count were significantly decreased ($p \le 0.01$ or $p \le 0.05$), while the number of abnormal sperm was significantly increased ($p \le 0.01$). In the exposed females, absolute live weight and body weight were significantly ($p \le 0.01$) lower than the corresponding values in control animals, while relative kidney and adrenal gland weights were above control values. The absolute kidney and adrenal gland weights and the relative liver weight were not affected. Histological examination of the exposed $F_1$-generation revealed slight atrophy of the seminiferous tubules in 7 out of 15 males. In addition, the number of mature sperm in the epididymis was reduced in 3 animals. In 13 of the 14 females, „fatty metamorphosis“ of the adrenal cortex was evident, marked by intracytoplasmic vacuoles in the epithelial cells. These effects were predominantly seen in the transitional area between the cortex and medulla. There was no effect on the kidneys, liver, prostate, ovaries, fallopian tubes, uterus or vagina, or on the oestrus cycle. Under these conditions, the no-effect-level for dams, embryos, foetuses and offspring was below 140 mg/kg body weight/day (NTP, 1986).

Rat embryos aged 9 1/2 days were incubated in vitro (in culture medium) for 48 hours. Malformations of the yolk sac, auditory pits, somites and neural groove were evident at concentrations of 1 mM methoxyacetic acid ($\hat{=}$90 µg/ml) and above. From 2 mM methoxyacetic acid ($\hat{=}$180 µg/ml), there was a significant decrease ($p \leq 0.05$) in the yolk sac diameter, the length from head to rump and the length of the skull. A reduced number of somites and decreased protein content in the embryo and yolk were also found. All of the embryos (n=24) were malformed at a concentration of 5 mM ($\hat{=}$451 µg/ml). In the control group (n=58), the figure was 8.6% (Rawling et al., 1985; Yonemoto et al., 1984).

Eleven-day-old embryos from CD-1 mice were incubated in culture medium for 6 hours with 2-methoxyacetic acid, with or without bovine serum. In the last hour ($^{3}$H)-thymidine was added and after 6 hours in total, DNA-synthesis was determined from thymidine incorporation. 2-Methoxyacetic acid inhibited DNA-synthesis dose-dependently in the serum-containing medium at concentrations of 5–100 mM (corresponding to 0.45–9 mg/ml), without affecting visible physiological functions (heart beat, yolk sac circulation). (A concentration of 5 mM is attained in embryos in vivo after a single administration to the dams of a teratogenic dose of 2-methoxyethanol.) The $ED_{50}$ was 25 mM (corresponding to 2.25 mg/ml). In the serum-free medium the $ED_{50}$ was only 5 mM (corresponding to 0.45 mg/ml). The addition of sodium acetate (5 mM) or sodium formate (1 mM) completely protected against the inhibitory action of 2-methoxyacetic acid in the serum-free mixture, whilst sarcosine (2 mM) was less effective in this respect. Sarcosine alone (5 mM) significantly inhibited thymidine incorporation, but this concentration produced severe embryotoxicity. According to the authors, the findings suggest that these substances, which also diminish the embryo- and foetotoxic effects in vivo, compete with the actions of methoxyacetic acid which inhibit DNA synthesis (Stedman and Welsch, 1989).

Sertoli germ cell cultures were prepared from the testes of 4-week-old rats. After incubation for 24–72 hours, methoxyacetic acid at a dose of around 1 mM ($\hat{=}$90 µg/ml) and above caused damage to spermatocytes at the pachytene stage. There was no effect on spermatocytes at the leptotene and zygotene stages, or on spermatogonia or Sertoli cells (Foster et al., 1984, 1986, 1987; Gray et al., 1985; Gray, 1986).

It has been suggested that decreased lactate synthesis in the Sertoli cells could be responsible for the disturbance in spermatogenesis. Methoxyacetic acid caused a significant decrease ($p \leq 0.05$) in lactate synthesis from 3 mM ($\hat{=}$270.3 µg/ml) in an in vitro study in Sertoli cells. The incubation periods were 6, 9 and 12 hours (Beattie et al., 1984).

7.9 Effects on the immune system

In a study on the immunotoxicological effects of methoxyacetic acid, female B6C3F1 mice (18–22 g) were given 25, 50 or 100 mg methoxyacetic acid/kg body weight/day by stomach tube for 2 weeks (5 days/week). Ten mice were used per group, including a control group. A significant ($p \leq 0.01$) decrease in thymus weight (by 48%) was seen from 50 mg/kg. Spleen and body weights were not affected. Methoxyacetic acid had no influence on the following parameters (6–8 animals were examined): number of cells in the spleen and the bone marrow, leucocyte and erythrocyte values, differential blood cell count, antibody plaque forming cell response (IgM antibodies), macrophage activity and host resistaqnce to *Listeria monocytogenes*. Cell-mediated immunity was studied using the proliferative reaction of spleen cells to T- and B-cells mitogens. The cytotoxicity to natural killer cells and cytotoxic T-lymphocyte-mediated cytolysis were also investigated. Apart from decreased thymus weight, no effects due to methoxyacetic acid were seen (House et al., 1985).

7.10 Neurotoxicity

No information available.

7.11 Other effects

Methoxyacetic acid inhibits respiration, oxidative phosphorylation and cytochrome c oxidase activity in rat liver microsomes and rat testis microsomes, at concentrations of about 300 µg/ml and above (Beattie and Brabec, 1986).

## 8. Experience in humans

No information available.

## 9. Threshold limit values

No information available.

## References


BASF AG, Gewerbehygiene und Toxikologie
Unpublished study (1981)

BASF AG
DIN-Sicherheitsdatenblatt (1986)

Beattie, P.J., Welsh, M.J., Brabec, M.J.
The effect of 2-methoxyethanol and methoxyacetic acid on sertoli cell lactate production and protein synthesis in vitro
Toxicol. Appl. Pharmacol., 76, 56–61 (1984)
see also: Effect of methoxyacetic acid on isolated sertoli cells
Fed. Proc., 43, 329 (1984)

Beattie, P.J., Brabec, M.J.
Methoxyacetic acid and ethoxyacetic acid inhibit mitochondrial function in vitro
J. Biochem. Toxicol., 1, 61–70 (1986)

Brown, N.A., Holt, D., Webb, M.
The teratogenicity of methoxyacetic acid in the rat
Toxicol. Lett., 22, 93–100 (1984)

Foster, P.M.D., Creasy, D.M., Foster, J.R., Thomas, L.V., Cook, M.W., Gangolli, S.D.
Testicular toxicity of ethylene glycol monomethyl and monoethyl ethers in the rat
Toxicol. Appl. Pharmacol., 69, 385–399 (1983)

Foster, P.M.D., Creasy, D.M., Foster, J.R., Gray, T.J.B.
Testicular toxicity produced by ethylene glycol monomethyl and monoethyl ethers in the rat
Environ. Health Perspect., 57, 207–217 (1984)

Foster, P.M.D., Blackburn, D.M., Moore, R.B., Lloyd, S.C.
Testicular toxicity of 2-methoxyacetaldehyde, a possible metabolite of ethylene glycol monomethyl ether, in the rat
Toxicol. Lett., 32, 73–80 (1986)

Foster, P.M.D., Lloyd, S.C., Blackburn, D.M.
Comparison of the in vivo and in vitro testicular effects produced by methoxy-, ethoxy-, and N-butoxyacetic acids in the rat
Toxicology, 43, 17–30 (1987)

Gray, T.J.B., Moss, E.J., Creasy, D.M., Gangolli, S.D.
Studies on the toxicity of some glycol ethers and alkoxyacetic acids in primary testicular cell cultures
Toxicol. Appl. Pharmacol., 79, 490–501 (1985)

Gray, T.J.B.
Testicular toxicity in vitro: sertoli-germ cell co-cultures as a model system
Food Chem. Toxicol., 24, 601–605 (1986)

House, R.V., Lauer, L.D., Murray, M.J., Ward, E.C., Dean, J.H.
Immunological studies in B6C3F1 mice following exposure to ethylene glycol monomethyl ether and its principal metabolite methoxyacetic acid
Toxicol. Appl. Pharmacol., 77, 358–362 (1985)

McGregor, D.B., Willins, M.J., McDonald, P., Holmström, H., McDonald, D., Niemeier, R.W.
Genetic effects of 2-methoxyethanol and bis(2-methoxyethyl)ether
Toxicol. Appl. Pharmacol., 70, 303–316 (1983)

Miller, R.R., Carreon, R.E., Young, J.T., McKenna, M.J.
Toxicity of methoxyacetic acid in rats
Fundam. Appl. Toxicol., 2, 158–160 (1982)

NTP (National Toxicology Program)
Methoxy acetic acid: reproduction and fertility assessment in CD-1 mice when administered in the drinking water
National Institute of Environmental Health Sciences, NTP-86-040 (1986)

Rawlings, S.J., Shuker, D.E.G., Webb, M., Brown, N.A.
The teratogenic potential of alkoxy acids in postimplantation rat embryo culture: structure-activity relationship
Toxicol. Lett., 28, 49–58 (1985)

Ritter, E.J., Scott, W.J., Randall, J.L., Ritter, J.M.
Teratogenicity of dimethoxyethyl phthalate and its metabolites methoxyethanol and methoxyacetic acid in the rat
Teratology, 32, 25–31 (1985)

Scott, W., Nau, H., Merker, H.J., Wittfoht, W.
Morphological investigations on the teratogenic effects of methoxyethanol in rat embryos
Teratology, 33, 29A–30A (1986)

Stedman, D.B., Welsch, F.
Inhibition of DNA synthesis in mouse whole embryo culture by 2-methoxyacetic acid and attenuation of the effects by simple physiological compounds
Toxicol. Lett., 45, 111–117 (1989)

Yonemoto, J., Brown, N.A., Webb, M.
Effects of dimethoxyethyl phthalate, monomethoxyethyl phthalate, 2-methoxyethanol and methoxyacetic acid in post implantation rat embryo in culture
Toxicol. Lett., 21, 97–102 (1984)

# o-Chlorobenzotrichloride

## 1. Summary and assessment

$LD_{50}$ values of 1380 and 2390 mg/kg body weight have been found for o-chlorobenzotrichloride following oral administration to rats. The observed symptoms point to an impairment of the nervous system.

The chemical is irritating to the conjunctiva and strongly irritating to the skin.

In vitro tests on *Salmonella typhimurium* and *Escherichia coli* have demonstrated mutagenic activity in two out of five strains of Salmonella. In a further in vitro test o-chlorobenzotrichloride has not induced point mutations at the HGPRT locus in V79 cells of Chinese hamsters whether metabolic activation has been used or not. The micronucleus test (in vivo), performed in mice, reveals a dose dependent induction of micronuclei in the bone marrow cells after single oral treatment with 100, 333 and 1000 mg/kg body weight respectively.

After long-term dermal application to the mouse (20 animals), the following tumours have been developed in the remaining 18 animals: one skin epithelioma, 4 lung adenocarcinomas and one fore-stomach carcinoma with metastases in the liver. On the basis of these results, a carcinogenic potential cannot be excluded for this chemical.

## 2. Name of substance

| | | |
|---|---|---|
| 2.1 | Usual name | o-Chlorobenzotrichloride |
| 2.2 | IUPAC-name | α,α,α,2-Tetrachlorotoluene |
| 2.3 | CAS-No. | 2136-89-2 |

## 3. Synonyms, common and trade names

2-Chloro-1-trichloromethylbenzene
α,α,α-Trichloro-2-chlorotoluene
α,α,α, 2-Tetrachlortoluol

## 4. Structural and molecular formulae

4.1 Structural formula

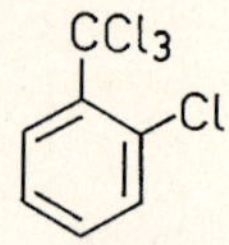

4.2 Molecular formula $C_7H_4Cl_4$

## 5. Physical and chemical properties

| | |
|---|---|
| 5.1 Molecular mass, g/mol | 229.9 |
| 5.2 Melting point, °C | 25 (freezing point) (Hoechst) |
| 5.3 Boiling point, °C | 264.3 (Weast, 1981) |
| 5.4 Vapour pressure, hPa | 0.1 (at 20 °C) (Bayer, 1989) |
| 5.5 Density, $g/cm^3$ | 1.515 (at 30 °C) (Hoechst)<br>1.458 (at 50 °C) (Bayer, 1989) |
| 5.6 Solubility in water | Poor; hydrolyses (Hoechst) |
| 5.7 Solubility in organic solvents | Ether, acetone (Weast, 1981) |
| 5.8 Solubility in fat | No information available |
| 5.9 pH-value | Acidic |
| 5.10 Conversion factor | 1 ppm $\hat{=}$ 9.41 $mg/m^3$<br>1 $mg/m^3$ $\hat{=}$ 0.11 ppm<br>(at 25 °C and 1013 hPa) |

## 6. Uses

Intermediate for use in the manufacture of dyestuffs and pesticides and in organic syntheses (Hoechst).

## 7. Experimental Results

7.1 Toxicokinetics and metabolism
No information available

7.2 Acute and subacute toxicity
o-Chlorobenzotrichloride is of low acute toxicity. The oral $LD_{50}$ in rats was 1380 mg/kg body weight (1270 mg/kg in males, 1490 mg/kg in females). The observed symptoms point to an impairment of the nervous system. Death occurred up to 17 days after exposure (Hoechst, 1987d).

In a further study on acute oral toxicity to rats, an $LD_{50}$ value of 2390 mg/kg body weight was reported (Bayer, 1980b).

In an inhalation risk test, 200 l air/hour were passed through about 50 g the test substance. Five male and 5 female rats were exposed to the enriched air for 7 hours in a 10 l glass chamber. The observation period was 14 days. All of the rats tolerated the 7-hour exposure without symptoms. No deaths occurred. When the rats were dissected at the end of the experiment, macroscopic examination revealed that the organs were physiologically normal (Bayer, 1980a).

## 7.3 Skin and mucous membrane effects

The application of 500 mg o-chlorobenzotrichloride to the dorsal skin of rabbits (treated area 2.5 × 2.5 cm) in the form of a paste led to clear skin irritation 24 and 72 hours after application. After 24 hours the skin had a grey-white coloration, and after 72 hours it had white to yellow blisters and marks. In addition, surface scurf and thickened, dry, flaking skin were observed (FhG, 1980a).

In a further study, 0.5 ml of the chemical was applied semi-occlusively to the backs of rabbits for 4 hours. One hour after the patch was removed, all of the animals had barely perceptible erythema and 2 of the rabbits had very slight oedema. Twenty four to 72 hours after the patch was removed the rabbits had barely perceptible to moderate erythema and barely perceptible to slight oedema. Seven days after application, a clear localized erythema was present in all animals and slight oedema was seen in 2 rabbits. In addition, 72 hours after removal of the patch, the skin was dry and chapped partly and had small areas of brown discoloration. Seven days after application the skin was scurfy and parchment-like and fine flakes were becoming detached. All of the effects were reversed 14 days after application. In this study, the substance proved to be irritating to the skin (Hoechst, 1987b).

In another study in rabbits, 0.5 g of the test sample was applied to a cellulose patch (2.5 × 2.5 cm) which was fixed to the hairless skin of one ear with adhesive tape for 1, 2, 4, 8 or 24 hours. The observation period lasted 7 days. The treated skin that was exposed for 1 or 2 hours was physiologically normal when the dressings were removed. Rabbits which were exposed for longer periods had moderate to very marked skin reddening and, when exposure was for 8 hours or more, slight to moderate swelling of the skin. The study revealed a strong skin-irritating effect (Bayer,1980a).

In a study designed to test the irritant effect of o-chlorobenzotrichloride on the eye, 100 µl of the substance was applied as a paste to the lower right eye lid of 6 rabbits. The untreated left eyes served as controls. The examination was carried out with an ophthalmoscope. To ascertain the effects on the cornea, a drop of fluorescein solution was applied directly to the cornea after 8 days, and the eye was examined under UV light with a cobalt blue filter. The results were recorded 24, 48 and 72 hours and 8 days after the beginning of the study. Evaluation of the results was carried out according to the scheme devised by Draize (1959). Neither the cornea nor the iris were damaged in any of the animals. Two of the 6 rabbits had slight intermittent reddening of the conjunctiva (grade 1) and 1 animal showed a slight swelling (grade 1). The results indicate that the substance is not an eye irritant in rabbits (FhG, 1980b).

In a further study, 0.1 ml of the chemical was instilled into the left conjunctival sac of each of 3 rabbits. The right eyes served as controls. The eyes were evaluated 1, 24, 48 and 72 hours after instillation. In addition, at 24 and 72 hours the corneas were examined for damage under UV light after instillation of a drop of 0.01% fluorescein sodium solution. The cornea and the iris were undamaged. The conjunctiva was markedly reddened after 1–24 hours and slightly red after 48 hours. Slight chemosis was present at 1 and 24 hours, an effect which was no longer apparent at 48 hours. This study demonstrated an irritant effect on the conjunctiva (Hoechst, 1987c).

o-Chlorobenzotrichloride was instilled into the conjunctival sac of 1 eye in each of 2 rabbits at a dose of 50 mg/rabbit. The untreated eyes served as controls. The observation period lasted 7 days. Moderate reddening and slight swelling of the conjuctiva were observed. Six days after exposure, the treated eyes were once again physiologically normal. This study showed that o-chlorobenzotrichloride was moderately irritating to the eye of the rabbit (Bayer, 1980a).

## 7.4 Sensitization

No information available.

## 7.5 Subchronic and chronic toxicity

No information available.

## 7.6 Genotoxicity

### 7.6.1 In vitro

o-Chlorobenzotrichloride was tested for point-mutagenic effects in *Salmonella typhimurium* strains TA 98, TA 100, TA 1535, TA 1537 and TA 1538 and in Escherichia coli WP2uvrA. The study was carried out with and without metabolic activation. The dose range used was 0.16 to 5000 μg test substance/plate. In the absence of metabolic activation o-chlorobenzotrichloride did not induce point mutations in any of the strains used. On addition of the metabolizing system an increase in the number of revertants was found in strains TA 98 and TA 100. o-Chlorobenzotrichloride therefore demonstrated point-mutagenic activity in this bacterial system in the presence of a metabolizing fraction (Hoechst, 1987a).

To investigate the potential of o-chlorobenzotrichloride inducing gene mutations at the HGPRT locus an in vitro test in V79 cells of Chinese hamsters was performed in two independent experiments, both with and without metabolic activation. The substance was tested with the following concentrations: without S9 mix: 2.0, 5.0, 10.0, 20.0, 30.0 and 40.0 μg/ml; with S9 mix: 4.0, 10.0, 20.0 and 40.0 μg/ml. According to the pre-experiment of toxicity the concentration ranges were selected to yield concentration related toxic effects. Up to the highest investigated concentration no relevant increase in mutant colony numbers was obtained whether metabolic activation was used or not. Therefore, o-chlorobenzotrichloride has to be considered to be non-mutagenic in this test (CCR, 1991a).

### 7.6.2 In vivo

A micronucleus test was performed to investigate the potential of o-chlorobenzotrichloride inducing micronuclei in polychromatic erythrocytes (PCE) in the bone marrow of the mouse. The test article was suspended in polyethylene glycol 400. This suspending agent was used as negative control. The volume administered orally was 10 ml/kg body weight (b. w.). 24 hours (h), 48 h and 72 h after a single application of the test article the bone marrow cells were collected for micronuclei analysis. Ten animals (5 male, 5 female) per test group were evaluated for the occurrence of micronuclei in PCEs, with the exception of the test article group at preparation interval 72 h in which only three males could be investigated because of lethalities. Per animal 1000 PCEs were scored for micronuclei. To describe a cytotoxic effect due to the treatment with the test article the ratio between polychromatic (PCE) and normochromatic erythrocytes (NCE) was determined in the same sample and reported as number of NCEs per 1000 PCEs. The following dose levels of the test article were tested: 24 h preparation interval 100, 333, and 1000 mg/kg b. w.; 48 h preparation interval 1000 mg/kg b.w.; 72 h preparation interval 1000 mg/kg b.w.. In a series of pre-experiments 1000 mg/kg b.w. was estimated to be the maximum tolerated dose. In comparison to the corresponding negative control there was a dose-dependent enhancement in the frequency of the detected micronuclei at preparation interval 24 h after treatment with the test article. Additionally, a statistically significant enhancement of the micronucleus frequencies after treatment with 1000 mg/kg b.w. o-chlorobenzotrichloride was observed at preparation intervals 24 h, 48 h, and 72 h. An appropriate reference mutagen was used as positive control which showed a distinct increase of induced micronucleus frequency. Under the experimental conditions reported, o-chlorobenzotrichloride did induce micronuclei and has therefore to be considered to be mutagenic in this micronucleus assay (CCR, 1991b).

## 7.7 Carcinogenicity

A preparation of o-chlorobenzotrichloride in benzene was applied to the shaved dorsal skin (shoulder blade) of 20 female mice (strain ICR-SLC, 7 weeks old) at a dose of 5 μl/mouse, twice a week for 30 weeks. The mice were then observed for a further 18 months. A control group of the same size (20 mice) was treated with 25 μl benzene in the same manner. The results of this long term study are summarized in the following table.

| Substance | Number of mice | Dose | Age at end of study (days) | Number of animals examined | Skin | Tumours Lungs | Gastro-intestinal tract |
|---|---|---|---|---|---|---|---|
| Benzene (control) | 20 | 25 μl | 551 | 17 | – | – | – |
| o-Chlorobenzotrichloride | 20 | 5 μl | 553 | 18 | 1[a] | 4[b] | 1[c] |

[a] Skin epithelioma
[b] Adenocarcinomas
[c] Fore stomach carcinoma with formation of metastases in the liver

Six out of 18 mice had malignant tumours, and 1 mouse had a benign tumour (not mentioned in the overview). No tumours of this type were seen in the controls. The authors interpreted this as a significant increase in the rate of tumour formation, even though this was clearly lower in comparison with p-chlorobenzotrichloride or benzotrichloride (Matsushita et al., 1977).

7.8 Reproductive toxicity

No information available.

7.9 Effects on the immune system

No information available.

7.10 Neurotoxicity

No information available.

7.11 Other effects

No information available.

## 8. Experience in humans

No information available.

## 9. Threshold limit values

No information available.

## References

Bayer AG, Institut für Toxikologie
o-Chlorbenzotrichlorid – Gewerbetoxikologische Untersuchungen
Unpublished Report No. 9064 (1980a)

Bayer AG, Institut für Toxikologie
o-Chlorbenzotrichlorid dest. – Untersuchung zur akuten oralen Toxizität an männlichen und weiblichen Wistar-Ratten
Unpublished Report (1980b)

Bayer AG
Safety data sheet (1989)

CCR (Cytotest Cell Research GmbH & Co. KG)
Gene mutation assay in Chinese hamster V79 cells in vitro with o-chlorobenzotrichloride
Projet 174824 (1991a)
Commisioned by BG Chemie

CCR (Cytotest Cell Research GmbH & Co. KG)
Micronucleus assay in bone marrow cells of the mouse with o-chlorobenzotrichloride
Project 174812 (1991b)
Commisioned by BG Chemie

FhG (Fraunhofer-Gesellschaft, Schmallenberg)
Prüfung von o-Chlorobenzotrichlorid auf primäre Hautreizwirkung
Bericht vom 24. 9. 1980a
Commissioned by Bayer AG

FhG (Fraunhofer-Gesellschaft, Schmallenberg)
Bericht über die Prüfung von o-Chlorobenzotrichlorid auf Schleimhautreizwirkung
Bericht vom 24. 9. 1980b
Commissioned by Bayer AG

Hoechst AG, Communication to BG Chemie

Hoechst AG, Pharma Forschung Toxicologie
o-Chlorbenzotrichlorid TTR – study of the mutagenic potential in strains of *Salmonella typhimurium* (Ames-Test) and *Escherichia coli*
Unpublished Report No. 87.0528 (1987a)

Hoechst AG, Pharma Forschung Toxikologie
o-Chlorbenzotrichlorid TTR – Prüfung auf Hautreizung am Kaninchen
Unpublished Report No. 87.0479 (1987b)

Hoechst AG, Pharma Forschung Toxikologie
o-Chlorbenzotrichlorid TTR – Prüfung auf Augenreizung am Kaninchen
Unpublished Report No. 87.0565 (1987c)

Hoechst AG, Pharma Forschung Toxikologie
o-Chlorbenzotrichlorid TTR – Prüfung der akuten Toxizität an der männlichen und weiblichen Wistar-Ratte
Unpublished Report No. 87.0566 (1987d)

Matsushita, H., Fukuda, K., Takemoto, K.
Carcinogenicity of benzotrichloride and its related compounds
Hoechst AG, Report No. 76/0729 (1977)

Weast, R.C. (ed.)
Handbook of Chemistry and Physics
62nd ed., p. C-166
CRC Press, Boca Raton, Florida (1981/1982)

# Diglycidyl ether

## 1. Summary and assessment

Diglycidyl ether (DGE) is acute toxic ($LD_{50}$ rats oral 450 mg/kg,rats dermal >1,000 mg/kg, $LC_{50}$ rats >200 ppm $\hat{=}$1.080 mg/m$^3$ air). A single administration, independent of the route, produces central nervous system depression and inhibits haematopoiesis and spermatogenesis. Subsequently, weight loss and leucopenia (followed by leucocytosis and haemoglobin reduction) are observed, though these effects are partially reversible. Damage to the kidneys, suprarenal glands, liver and lungs is also described.

In sub-acute toxicity tests, comparable but more marked effects are seen. After repeated dermal application (from 30 mg/kg) and intravenous injection (from 12.5 mg/kg), leucopenia occurs, with depression of the bone marrow and damage to the liver and testes. Necrosis in the kidney marrow and haemorrhages in the suprarenal glands are also described, as well as focal lymphoid necroses and thymus atrophy. Sub-chronic inhalation exposure (from 3 ppm $\hat{=}$ 16.2 mg/m$^3$) also produces pulmonary oedema, obstruction of the lung and pneumonia.

DGE has strong local irritant and corrosive effects. Depending on the concentration, even a single application to the skin, the eyes or the mucous membranes of the respiratory and/or gastro-intestinal tracts can lead to degenerative tissue damage, with erythema, oedema, haemorrhage and necrosis, effects which are more marked with repeated application.

DGE is a skin sensitiser in guinea-pigs.

In the Salmonella/microsome test, DGE is mutagenic in the TA 100 strain both with and without S9 mix, whilst the corresponding test with the TA 98 strain is negative. The substance also displays mutagenic activity in conidia of *Neurospora*, and produces chromosomal aberrations in root tips of *Vicia faba*.

In a poorly-documented study on the long-term toxicity of DGE, malignant skin tumours are described following repeated dermal treatment, their incidence increasing in line with the dosage. The first tumour appeared in the fifth month of the study.

The present findings indicate that DGE may be a potential carcinogen. For this reason, since 1980 DGE has been in Section III B of the German list of MAK-values.

## 2. Name of substance

| | | |
|---|---|---|
| 2.1 | Usual name | Diglycidyl ether |
| 2.2 | IUPAC-name | Bis(2,3-epoxypropyl)-ether |
| 2.3 | CAS-No. | 2238-07-5 |

## 3. Synonyms, common and trade names

Di(2,3-epoxypropyl)ether
DGE

## 4. Structural and molecular formulae

4.1 Structural formula

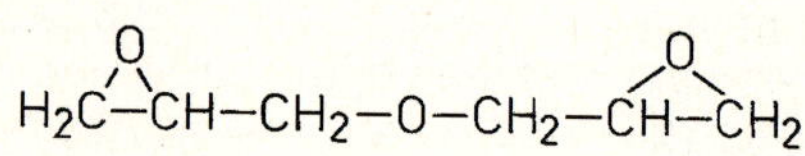


4.2 Molecular formula $C_6H_{10}O_3$

## 5. Physical and chemical properties

| | | |
|---|---|---|
| 5.1 | Molecular mass, g/mol | 130.16 |
| 5.2 | Melting point, °C | No information available |
| 5.3 | Boiling point, °C | 260 (Hine et al., 1981) |
| 5.4 | Vapour pressure, hPa | 0.12 (at 20 °C) (Hine et al., 1981) |
| 5.5 | Density, g/cm$^3$ | 1.1195 (Hine et al., 1981) |
| 5.6 | Solubility in water | No information available |
| 5.7 | Solubility in organic solvents | No information available |
| 5.8 | Solubility in fat | No information available |
| 5.9 | pH-value | – |
| 5.10 | Conversion factor | 1 ppm $\hat{=}$ 5.40 mg/m$^3$<br>1 mg/m$^3$ $\hat{=}$ 0.19 ppm<br>(at 25 °C and 1013 hPa) |

## 6. Uses

By-product in the manufacture of epichlorohydrin (Hine et al., 1981).

## 7. Experimental results

### 7.1 Toxicokinetics and metabolism

No information available

### 7.2 Acute and subacute toxicity

**Table 1.** Studies on acute oral toxicity

| Species | Oral $LD_{50}$ (10-day observation period) (mg/kg) |
|---|---|
| Rat | 450 (10% in propylene glycol) |
| Rat | 510 (neat) |
| Mouse | 170 (10% in propylene glycol) |
| Mouse | 192 (10% in propylene glycol) |

Lower doses of DGE cause slight dyspnoea and depression of the central nervous system (CNS); higher doses lead to more serious depression of the CNS, resulting in prostration, lying on the side, shock, coma and death. Autopsy revealed haemorrhages in the lungs, hyperaemia and irritation of the gastro-intestinal tract, effects on the liver and kidneys, and inflammation of the adrenal glands (Hine et al., 1956, 1981).

The intravenous $LD_{50}$ in the rabbit is 141 mg/kg. Autopsy revealed severe congestion of the lungs, ischaemia of the liver and kidneys, and ascites (Hine et al., 1956, 1981).

A significant, dose-dependent decrease in the number of leukocytes and polymorphonuclear cells occurred on intravenous injection of DGE to groups of three New Zealand rabbits at doses of 50, 100 and 200 mg/kg. There were no deaths at 50 and 100 mg/kg. At 200 mg/kg, two rabbits died after 2 days, and one after 3 days. An increased number of nucleated erythrocytes was observed in the peripheral blood at 100 mg/kg (Hine et al., 1961).

The following $LD_{50}$ values were found on dermal application:

**Table 2**

| Species | $LD_{50}$ (mg/kg) |
|---|---|
| Rabbit | 1500 (approximate) |
| Rabbit | >1000 |
| Rat | >1000 |

In both species the animals developed severe skin irritation and systemic effects similar to those seen on intravenous injection. Depression of the CNS, weight loss and leukopenia were observed 3 days after application, which developed into leukocytosis over the following days. In addition, a reduction in the haemoglobin concentration occurred in the rabbit (Hine et al., 1956,1961).

The following $LC_{50}$ values were reported in acute inhalation toxicity tests:

**Table 3**

| Species | Exposure time (hours) | ppm | $LC_{50}$ | mg/$m^3$ air |
|---|---|---|---|---|
| Rabbit | 24 | 13.3 | | 71.8 |
| Mouse | 4 | 86 | | 464.4 |
| Rat | 4 | >200 | | >1080.0[a] |
| Mouse | 8 | 30 | | 162.0 |
| Rat | 8 | 68 | | 367.2 |
| Mouse | 4 | 30 | (24–37) | 162.0 |
| Rat | 8 | >200 | | >1080.0[a] |

[a] Highest attainable concentration

The immediate effect of exposure was irritation of the mucous membranes; however, within 24 hours the animals showed depression of the CNS, clouding of the cornea and iritation of the skin and mucous membranes. High concentrations (113 ppm) caused dyspnoea. At autopsy, lung congestion and enlargement of the kidneys and adrenal glands were seen (Hine et al., 1956).

On exposure of rabbits to 3, 6, 12 and 24 ppm for 24 hours, leukocytosis was seen only at the highest concentration; irritation of the mucous membranes was evident from 3 ppm and increased with increasing dose (Hine et al., 1961).

In further studies, DGE was applied dermally at 0.5 or 1.0 g/kg to groups of five male Long-Evans rats (weight 115–145 g). A significant dose-related decrease in leukocytes occurred after 3 days in both groups, whilst the number of bone-marrow cells remained unchanged. No deaths were observed. Severe skin irritation was seen in one animal and pneumonia in another (Hine et al., 1961).

After a single application of 1.13 g/kg DGE to the shaved dorsal skin of male New Zealand rabbits (weight 1.9–4.2 kg), a significant reduction ($p < 0.001$) was found in the number of leukocytes and in the haemoglobin level on the sixth day of the investigation. All rabbits showed weight loss. A few hours after the application, skin oedema with subsequent induration and staining of the skin occurred (Hine et al., 1961).

Groups of three rabbits were exposed by inhalation to 3, 6, 12 and 24 ppm for 24 hours. At 3 or 6 ppm, body weight was unaffected and there were no notable effects on the peripheral blood. A concentration of 12 ppm led to an increase in platelets and 24 ppm led to an increase in leukocytes, particularly polymorphonuclear cells. At these concentrations, two animals died on day 5 of the investigation and a third on day 7, with distinct weight loss. On pathomorphological examination, there were inflammatory changes in the lungs and liver and haemorrhages in the kidneys and lungs. A distinct atrophy of the testes was reported (without detailed data; Hine et al., 1981).

Acute intramuscular injection of 25 mg/kg in three dogs led to severe local oedema with subsequent abscess-formation. No evaluation of blood parameters was possible because of the severe inflammatory reaction (Hine et al., 1961).

The results of investigations into the subacute toxicity of DGE are summarized in Table 4.

After repeated application by various routes, severe inflammatory and necrotic effects on the skin and mucous membranes occurred, as well as damage to the bone marrow, peripheral blood (leukopenia), testes and thymus. At higher doses, liver and kidney

**Table 4.** Studies on the subacute toxicity of DGE

| Species | Strain | Sex | Number of animals per group | Route of exposure | Individual dose | Treatment schedule | Duration of study | Results (toxic effects) |
|---|---|---|---|---|---|---|---|---|
| Rabbit | California Albino | ♂ | 6 | Dermal | 0.2 ml/ animal | Daily | Until occurrence of massive local or systemic effects | Weight loss severe skin irritation with erythema and oedema |
| Rat | Long Evans | ♂ | 5 | Dermal | 15–125 mg/kg | 20 applica tions | 4 weeks[a] | None (15 mg) from 30 mg: weight loss, decrease in polymorphonuclear cells in blood necrosis of the skin, clouding of the cornea, leukopenia, generalised aplasia of the bone marrow, thymus atrophy, focal lymphoid necroses, necrosis of the proximal convoluted tubules of the kidneys, focal necroses in the testes, haemorrhages of the adrenal medulla |
| Rat | Long Evans | | | Dermal | 250 and 500 mg/kg | 6 applications | 2 weeks[b] | |

| | | | | | | | | |
|---|---|---|---|---|---|---|---|---|
| Rabbit | New Zealand | ♂ | 3 | Injection (i.v.) in propylene glycol | 25 mg/kg | 4 applications | 4 weeks | Slight leukopenia, decrease in polymorphonuclear cells |
| Dog | Mongrel | ♂ | 3 | Injection (i.v.) in physiological saline | 12.5 mg/kg | 7 applications | No data | Leukopenia, necrosis at the site of injection |
| Dog | Mongrel | ♂ | 3 | Injection (i.v.) in physiological saline | 25 mg/kg | 2–3 applications | Not given | 2 of 3 animals died after 6 and 7 days, pneumonia, haemorrhages and necrosis of the liver, leukopenia |

[a] Survived
[b] Two out of five died

damage was also observed. Repeated dermal application of 15 mg DGE/kg body weight is tolerated without effect and thus represents a "no effect level" for this route of exposure (Hine et al., 1956, 1961).

7.3 Skin and mucous membrane effects

Acute and repeated application to the intact or abraded skin of rabbits caused severe irritation and corrosion. Repeated application also caused necrosis of the deeper lying tissues (Hine et al., 1981).

Undiluted DGE and a 15% solution in propylene glycol caused severe irritation and corneal necrosis on instillation into the eyes (Hine et al., 1981).

Inhalation exposure of male white rabbits to 20–27 ppm DGE for 4 hours caused complete detachment of the corneal epithelium from the stroma and damage to the stroma. The regeneration rate of the epithelium and its dehydrogenase activity remained unaffected (Mettier et al., 1962).

7.4 Sensitization

DGE is strongly sensitizing in guinea-pigs (without further details; Hine et al., 1981).

7.5 Subchronic and chronic toxicity

The results of studies on subchronic inhalation toxicity in rats are given in Table 5.

On exposure to 3 or 20 ppm the observed range of effects correspond to those seen after subacute dermal or intravenous administration, while exposure to 0.3 ppm over a substantially longer period gives rise to only marginal changes to the germinal epithelium.

7.6 Genotoxicity

7.6.1 In vitro

In the Salmonella/microsome test on strains TA 98 and TA 100, DGE shows dose-dependent mutagenic activity in strain TA 100 in the dose range 0.01–0.5 mg/plate, both with and without metabolic activation (S9 mix from rat liver, no further information). A dose of 10 mg DGE/plate was bacteriotoxic (Wade et al., 1976, 1978).

The mutagenic activity of DGE was also tested in *Neurospora* W40 "distinctus", by measuring the number of adenine-deficient revertants. DGE was mutagenic in this test (no further details; Kölmark and Westergaard, 1953).

DGE causes chromosomal aberrations in *Vicia faba* root tips (no further details; Ehrenberg and Hussain, 1981).

**Table 5.** Studies on the subchronic toxicity of DGE

| Species | Strain | Sex | Number of animals per group | Route of exposure | Individual dose | Treatment schedule | Duration of study | Results (toxic effects) |
|---|---|---|---|---|---|---|---|---|
| Rat | Long Evans | ♂ | 30 | Inhalation | 0.3 ppm[a] | 4 hours/day 5 days/week max. 60 exposures over 90 days | 52 weeks | Focal degeneration of the germinal epithelium |
| Rat | Long Evans | ♂ | 30 | Inhalation | 3.0 ppm[a] | 4 hours/day 5 days/week 19 exposures over 29 days | 52 weeks | Lung infections, peribronchiolitis, weight loss, depression of the haematopoietic system, fatty dystrophy of the liver, necrosis of the seminiferous tubules |
| Rat | Long Evans | ♂ | 30 | Inhalation | 20 ppm[a] | 4 hours 3 or 4 exposures | 52 weeks | 3 out of 30 animals died after 3 and 4 exposures, oedema and congestion of the lungs, weight loss, leukopenia, depression of the bone marrow |

[a] Nominal concentration

7.6.2 In vivo
No information available.

7.7 Carcinogenicity
McCammon et al. (1957) and Kotin and Falk (1963) reported a study on the long-term effects of DGE, but the experiment was insufficiently documented and only capable of producing limited results. The test substance was applied dermally three times a week to C57B1 mice (of unspecified sex). Groups of 20 animals received a total dose of ca. 98 mg or 33 mg. In the higher dose group, four of the ten surviving animals developed malignant skin tumours, the first of which appeared after 5 months. In the lower dose group, one out of eight animals had a skin tumour. No further details were provided of the experimental methods, the evaluation of the results, or the histology of the observed tumours.

7.8 Reproductive toxicity
No information available.

7.9 Effects on the immune system
No information available.

7.10 Neurotoxicity
See 7.2.

7.11 Other effects
No information available.

## 8. Experience in humans

No information available.

## 9. Threshold limit values

AK-value 0.6 mg/m$^3$ air category IIIb (DFG, 1980).

## References

DFG (Deutsche Forschungsgemeinschaft)
Mitteilung XVI der Senatskommission zur Prüfung gesundheitsschädlicher Arbeitstoffe
Verlag Chemie, Weinheim (1980)

Ehrenberg, L., Hussain, S.
Genetic toxicity of some important epoxides
Mutat. Res., 86, 1–113 (1981)

Hine, C., Kodama, J.K., Wellington, J.S., Dunlap, M.K., Anderson, K.H.
The toxicology of glycidol and some glycidyl ethers
Arch. Ind. Health, 14, 250–264 (1956)

Hine, C., Kodama, J.K., Guzman, R.J., Dunlap, M.K., Lima, R., Loquvam, G.S.
Effects of diglycidylether on blood of animals
Arch. Environ. Health, 2, 31–50 (1961)

Hine, C., Rowe, V.K., White, E.R., Darmer, K.I., Youngblood, G.T.
Epoxy compounds
In: Clayton, G.D., Clayton F.E. (eds.)
Patty's Industrial Hygiene and Toxicology
3rd ed., Vol. 2A, p. 2204
John Wiley and Sons, New York (1981)

Kölmark, G., Westergaard, M.
Further studies on chemically induced reversions at the adenine locus of neurospora
Hereditas, 39, 209–224 (1953)

Kotin, P., Falk, H.L.
Organic peroxides, hydrogen peroxides, epoxides and neoplasia
Radiat. Res., Suppl. 3, 193–211 (1963)

McCammon, C.J., Kotin, P., Falk, H.L.
The cancerogenic potency of certain diepoxides
Proc. Am. Assoc. Cancer Res., 229–230 (1957)

Mettier, S.R., Boyer, H.K., McEwen, W.K., Ivanhoe, F., Meyers, F.H., Hine, C.
Effects of air pollutant mixtures on the eye
Arch. Environ. Health, 4, 103–107 (1962)

Wade, M.J., Moyer, J.W., Hine, C.
The mutagenicity of epoxides
Fed. Proc. Fed. Am. Soc. Exp. Biol., 35, 504 (1976)

Wade, M.J., Moyer, J.W., Hine, C.
Mutagenic action of a series of epoxides
Mutat. Res., 66, 367–371 (1979)

# p-Chlorobenzotrichloride

## 1. Summary and assessment

Up to 96% of a single oral dose of p-chlorobenzotrichloride is metabolized and eliminated within 4–6 days, 87% being excreted in the urine and 9% in the faeces. The remaining 4% is found in the tissues. 4-Chlorohippuric acid appears as the main metabolite (>90%) in the urine. In the faeces, the metabolites 4-chlorobenzoic acid and $\alpha,\alpha',4,4'$-tetrachlorostilbene have been found.

The chemical appears to be of low acute oral toxicity ($LD_{50}$ rat oral 614–1350 mg/kg; rat dermal 1900 mg/kg). On inhalation it is clearly toxic ($LC_{50}$ rat and mouse 125 mg/m$^3$). Moreover, it is rapidly absorbed through the skin. The toxic symptoms after acute administration (impairment of posture and motor functions, reduced reflex reactions, spasms and dyspnoea) are due to an effect on the central nervous system. On anatomical/pathological examination, the chemical causes changes in the internal organs, predominantly the liver (signs of dystrophy in the lobules) and the lungs (bronchitis and bronchopneumonia).

p-Chlorobenzotrichloride causes marked irritation of the skin, less marked irritation of the mucous membranes, and skin sensitization.

On repeated oral administration (Lim-test), a cumulative effect is observed, which is reduced in the prolonged elimination phase of the chemical. In rats and guinea-pigs exposed repeatedly by inhalation for 4 months, weight loss and functional disturbances of the nervous system, liver, kidneys, lungs and blood occur. At a concentration of 9.67 mg/m$^3$ air, morphological changes have been identified in the lungs (bronchitis, focal pneumonia and bleeding in the alveoli), in the nervous system (pyknosis of the large neurones, neurones with central chromatolysis, vacuolization of the cytoplasm) and in the liver (anisocaryocytosis of the hepatocytes, focal leukocyte infiltration). This exposure level may be lethal after 1 month. The medium and low concentrations (1.72 and 0.1 mg/m$^3$ air, respectively) lead intermittently to functional disturbances (no further details).

The chemical has a dose-dependent point-mutagenic effect in the Salmonella/microsome test in strain TA 98, and also to a lesser extent in strains TA 100 and TA 1537, independent of whether S9 mix is added or not. In the HGPRT test with Chinese hamster V79 cells in vitro, a point-mutagenic effect is evident.

On repeated oral administration in long-term tests in mice, a dose-dependent carcinogenic effect is seen. Carcinogenic activity has also been observed on repeated dermal application in long-term studies.

On the basis of the findings from subchronic inhalation studies, a Russian TLV of 0.01 mg/m$^3$ air has been established, with the risk phrases "penetrates the skin, dangerous substance class I".

## 2. Name of substance

| | | |
|---|---|---|
| 2.1 | Usual name | p-Chlorobenzotrichloride |
| 2.2 | IUPAC-name | α,α,α,4-Tetrachlorotoluene |
| 2.3 | CAS-No. | 5216-25-1 |

## 3. Synonyms, common and trade names

4-Chloro-1-trichloro-methylbenzene
α,α,α-Trichloro-4-chlorotoluene
4-Chlorobenzotrichloride
p-Chlorbenzotrichlorid

## 4. Structural and molecular formulae

4.1 Structural formula

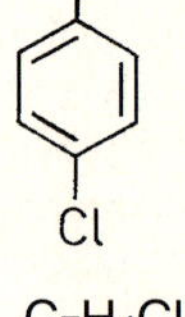


4.2 Molecular formula $C_7H_4Cl_4$

## 5. Physical and chemical properties

| | | |
|---|---|---|
| 5.1 | Molecular mass, g/mol | 229.9 |
| 5.2 | Melting point, °C | 4.0 (Hoechst, 1989) |
| 5.3 | Boiling point, °C | 240 (Hoechst, 1989) |
| 5.4 | Vapour pressure, hPa | 0.04 (at 20 °C) (Hoechst, 1989) |
| 5.5 | Density, $g/cm^3$ | 1.49 (at 20 °C) (Hoechst, 1989) |
| 5.6 | Solubility in water | Poorly soluble, hydrolyes (Hoechst, 1989) |
| 5.7 | Solubility in organic solvents | Miscible with all common solvents (Hoechst, 1989) |
| 5.8 | Solubility in fat | No information available |
| 5.9 | pH-value | No information available |
| 5.10 | Conversion factor | 1 ppm $\hat{=}$ 9.41 $mg/m^3$<br>1 $mg/m^3$ $\hat{=}$ 0.106 ppm<br>(at 25 °C and 1013 hPa) |

## 6. Uses

Intermediate in the manufacture of herbicides, pharmaceuticals, dyestuffs and disinfectants (Chalepo et al., 1984; Quistad et al., 1985; Hoechst, 1989).

## 7. Experimental results

7.1 Toxicokinetics and metabolism

$^{14}$C-Ring-labelled 4-chlorobenzotrichloride was administered orally to fasted female Sprague-Dawley albino rats (weight 166–168 g) as a single dose by stomach tube. The doses used were 1.5 mg/kg (2 animals, radioactivity ca. 5 μCi) and 102 mg/kg (1 animal, radioactivity ca. 38 μCi), administered in 0.5 ml rapeseed oil. The animals were kept in metabolic cages for 4–6 days. The urine, faeces and $CO_2$ from the exhaled air were collected daily. The animals were killed after 4 or 6 days. The dissected tissues were weighed, appropriately treated, and frozen for analytical evaluation. Metabolites were quantitatively and qualitatively determined. The following results were reported:

| | % of administered dose of 4-chlorobenzotrichloride | |
|---|---|---|
| | after 6 days (1.5 mg/kg) | after 4 days (102 mg/kg) |
| Urine | 87 | 77 |
| Faeces | 9 | 14 |
| Carcass | 4 | 4 |
| $CO_2$ | <0.02 | – |
| Volatile organic substances | <0.002 | – |
| Total | 100 | 95 |

| | % $^{14}C$-labelled metabolites analysed in the urine | | | | |
|---|---|---|---|---|---|
| | 1.5 mg/kg | | | | 102 mg/kg |
| Days | 1 | 2 | 3 | 4–6 | 1 |
| 4-Chlorobenzotrichloride | <0.3 | <0.9 | – | – | <0.4 |
| 4-Chlorobenzoic acid | 0.7 | 4 | 6 | 9 | 5 |
| 4-Chlorohippuric acid | 96 | 37 | 27 | 8 | 88 |
| Thin layer chromatogram, start zone contains glucuronide[a] | 4 | 59 | 64 | 73 | 3 |

[a] Not analysed

| | % $^{14}C$-labelled metabolites analysed in the faeces | | |
|---|---|---|---|
| | 1.5 mg/kg | 102 mg/kg | |
| Days | 1 | 1 | 2 |
| $CH_3CN$ extract | 28 | 38 | 64 |
| 4-Chlorobenzotrichloride | <0.3 | 1 | 1 |
| 4-Chlorobenzoic acid | 10 | 7 | 6 |
| $\alpha$, $\alpha'$,4, 4'-Tetrachlorostilbene | 8 | 13 | 13 |
| Remaining solids | 72 | 62 | 36 |

It was concluded that most of the radioactivity excreted in the faeces was not excreted in the form of the above metabolites (Quistad et al., 1985).

7.2 Acute and subacute toxicity

p-Chlorobenzotrichloride is of low acute oral and dermal toxicity to rats, with an oral LD50 of between 614 and 1350 mg/kg body weight (Chalepo et al., 1984; Bayer, 1980a; Hoechst, 1984), and a dermal LD50 in female rats of 1900 mg/kg body weight. In preliminary studies, male rats appeared not to be more sensitive (Hoechst, 1988a).

Acute inhalation exposure was clearly toxic, the $LC_{50}$ value being 125 mg/m$^3$ air in rats and mice (Chalepo et al., 1984).

No deaths were seen in an inhalation risk test in which 200 l air/hour were passed through about 50 g of the test substance and groups of male and female rats were exposed to the enriched air for 7 hours. The treatment was tolerated without symptoms (Bayer, 1980a).

Prominent symptoms following acute exposure were postural effects, impaired reflexes and breathing difficulties. In addition, muscle spasms occurred on inhalation exposure. At autopsy, the main effects were seen in the liver (lesions, dystrophic changes), but bronchitis and early signs of bronchopneumonia were also evident in the lungs.

7.3 Skin and mucous membrane effects

The substance had a marked local effect on the skin, causing dermatitis which cleared up only slowly (no further details). A slight irritant effect was seen on direct application of the chemical to the conjunctiva in rabbits (no further details; Chalepo et al., 1984).

In a patch test, 500 µl of the liquid chemical was applied to the shaved dorsal skin of 6 male albino rabbits (white New Zealand, weight 2.14 kg) for 24 hours. The application was occlusive. Within 24 hours the skin had a white coloration and a superficial, whitish scab had formed over the treated area. After 8 days the skin was dried out and slightly brown. Thus the chemical was corrosive to rabbit skin (Schreiber, 1980a).

To test the irritant effect on the eye, 100 µl of the liquid chemical was instilled into the right conjuctival sac of each of 6 male albino rabbits (white New Zealand, weight 2.1 kg).

The untreated left eyes served as controls. The eyes were examined 24, 48 and 72 hours and 8 days later. Slight reversible cloudiness of the cornea was seen. The iris was not affected. The conjunctiva was slightly red and slight chemosis and secretion were observed, which cleared up during the 8-day observation period. The substance was thus slightly irritating to the eye (Schreiber, 1980b).

7.4 Sensitization

The chemical had a clear sensitizing effect on the skin in an epicutaneous test in guinea-pigs. In the course of the study, a 1% solution was applied to the skin 10 times, followed by a challenge with a 1% solution, which caused skin-sensitization effects in 60% of the animals (no further details; Chalepo et al., 1984).

7.5 Subchronic and chronic toxicity

In a subchronic inhalation study, rats and guinea-pigs were exposed to p-chlorobenzotrichloride for 4 months (daily exposure duration not specified) at concentrations of 9.67, 1.72 and 0.1 mg/m$^3$ air. After 1 month's exposure at 9.67 mg/m$^3$ air, the rats were severely emaciated and showed pronounced functional disturbances of the nervous system, liver, kidneys and blood (no further details). Morphological changes were seen in the lungs (purulent destructive bronchitis, focal pneumonia and alveolar bleeding), in the nervous system (in the cerebral cortex, pyknosis of the large neurons, isolated neurons with central chromatolysis and vacuolisation of the cytoplasm) and in the liver (anisocaryocytosis of the hepatocytes and slight, focal leukocyte infiltration). Some of the animals died, and exposure was therefore discontinued. The concentration of 1.72 mg/m$^3$ air caused temporary body weight reduction and affected the nervous system (phasic effects on the functional condition of the central and peripheral systems). Morphological changes to the cerebral cortex and the brain stem were moderate and transitory (not further described). Effects on the respiratory system included a decrease in breathing frequency and a reduction in the volume breathed per minute. There were morphological changes in the lungs (moderate hyperplasia of the lymphatic system in the lumen of the bronchi and the vessels, indications of hypertrophy of the bronchial epithelia, an increase in the diameter of the bronchioli and focal emphysema). During a recovery period (duration not specified) the adverse effects proved to be reversible. Repeated exposure to 0.1 mg/m$^3$ air led to temporary functional disturbances (not further described), which were not present at the end of the study. There were no morphological correlations. The authors therefore considered 0.1 mg/m$^3$ air to be the threshold concentration (Chalepo et al., 1984).

## 7.6 Genotoxicity

### 7.6.1 In vitro

p-Chlorobenzotrichloride was tested for point-mutagenic effects in *Salmonella typhimurium* strains TA 98, TA 100, TA 1535, TA 1537 and TA 1538 and in *Escherichia coli* WP2uvrA. The study was carried out with and without a metabolizing system (liver homogenate from Aroclor-treated rats). Based on studies on bacteriotoxicity, 7 different doses ranging from 0.16 to 500 µg/plate were tested. The chemical had a point-mutagenic effect in strain TA 98, whether or not S9-mix was added. There were also signs of a point-mutagenic effect in strains TA 100 and TA 1537, with or without S9-mix. p-Chlorobenzotrichloride was therefore assessed as being mutagenic (Hoechst, 1986).

A point-mutagenic effect was also found in an HGPRT test in Chinese hamster V79 cells in vitro, with and without metabolic activation (S9-mix). The doses used were as follows: without S9-mix, 100, 200, 300, and 500 µg/ml; with S9-mix, 100, 300, 500, 750, and 850 µg/ml. In the presence of S9-mix, a significant increase in the number of mutated colonies and in the mutation frequency was seen at 500 µg/ml and above. No mutagenic activity was evident without S9-mix (no further details; Hoechst, 1988b).

### 7.6.2 In vivo

No information available.

## 7.7 Carcinogenicity

Groups of 30 female mice (8 weeks old, ICR strain) were given p-chlorobenzotrichloride by stomach tube twice weekly for 17.5 weeks. The following doses were administered in 0.1 ml sesame oil: 0.05, 0.13, 0.32, 0.8, and 2 µl/mouse. The entire experiment lasted 18 months. The number and distribution of observed tumours is shown in Table 1. The first tumours observed were thymus tumours and malignant lympho-adenomas. From about 5 months, squamous epithelial carcinomas developed in the fore-stomach. Lung tumours occurred most frequently, with the following incidences: 5/22 at 0.05 µl, 8/28 at 0.13 µl, 16/22 at 0.32 µl, 25/29 at 0.8 µl, and 19/29 at 2 µl. In addition, skin cancer, breast cancer and cancer of the salivary glands were observed (Fukuda et al., 1979).

p-Chlorobenzotrichloride (5µl) in benzene was applied to the shaved dorsal skin (shoulder blade) of 22 female mice (7 weeks old, CR-SLC strain) twice weekly for 30 weeks. The mice were subsequently observed for up to 9 months. A control group of 20 female

**Table 1.** Tumours in female mice following chronic oral administration of p-chlorobenzotrichloride

| Group/<br>Dose (μl/animal) | A<br>2 | B<br>0.8 | C<br>0.32 | D<br>0.13 | E<br>0.05 | Control |
|---|---|---|---|---|---|---|
| Number of animals/group | 29 | 29 | 22 | 28 | 22 | 26 |
| Average survival time[h] | 6.2 | 14.8 | 16.9 | 16.9 | 17.9 | 17.5 |
| Tumours | | | | | | |
| Fore-stomach | | | | | | |
| Squamous epithelial carcinomas | 7 | 6 | – | – | – | – |
| Carcinomas in situ | 3 | 4 | 1 | – | – | – |
| Multiple papillomas | 1 | 2 | 4 | 3 | 2 | – |
| Glandular stomach carcinomas | – | – | – | – | 1 | – |
| Lungs | | | | | | |
| Adenocarcinomas | 2 | 15 | 10 | 7 | 3 | – |
| Multiple adenomas | 17 | 10 | 6 | 1 | 2 | 1 |
| Malignant lymphomas | 5 | – | – | 1 | – | 1 |
| Skin tumours | 6[a] | 2[b,c] | 1b | – | – | – |
| Other tumours | 1[d] | 3[e] | 1[f] | 1[g] | – | – |
| Number of animals with tumours | | | | | | |
| Malignant | 16 | 20 | 10 | 8 | 4 | 1 |
| Benign | 9 | 7 | 7 | 2 | 2 | 1 |
| Total | 25/29 | 27/29 | 17/22 | 10/28 | 6/22 | 2/26 |

[a] Squamous epithelium
[b] Spindle cell sarcoma
[c] Sweat gland carcinoma
[d] Mammary adenocarcinoma
[e] Squamous epithelial carcinoma in the auditory canal, 2 salivary gland adenocarcinomas
[f] Granulosa cell tumour of the ovary
[g] Benign stomach cell carcinoma in situ
[h] Average survival time is expressed in months after the end of administration

**Table 2.** Tumour incidence following repeated dermal application of p-chlorobenzotrichloride (A) and benzene (control) (B) in a long-term study

| Substance | A | B |
|---|---|---|
| Dose/mouse | 5μl | 25 μl |
| Number of applications/week | 2 | 1 |
| Application period (weeks) | 30 | 30 |
| Number of animals | 22 | 20 |
| Study duration in days | 278 | 551 |
| Tumours | | |
| Skin | | |
| Squamous epithelial carcinoma | 12 | 0 |
| Sarcoma | 2 | 0 |
| Papilloma | 2 | 0 |
| Lung carcinoma | 1 | 0 |
| Oesophageal carcinoma | 5 | 0 |
| Fore-stomach carcinoma | 2 | 0 |
| Leukaemia | 1 | 0 |
| Thymus tumours | 1 | 0 |
| Number of animals with tumours | | |
| Malignant | 16 | 0 |
| Benign | 2 | 0 |
| Total | 18/22 | 0/20 |

mice received weekly applications of 25 μl benzene/mouse in the same manner as the treated animals. The results are shown in Table 2. The authors considered that the tumorigenic effect of p-chlorobenzotrichloride following oral or dermal application was comparable with that of benzotrichloride (Matsushita et al., 1977).

7.8 Reproductive toxicity

No information available.

7.9 Effects on the immune system

No information available.

7.10 Neurotoxicity

See chapter 7.5.

7.11 Other effects

In the Lim-test (short-term test for cumulative effects) a factor of 1.6 was reported following repeated administration by stomach tube. This indicated that the chemical had a marked cumulative effect (no further details; Chalepo et al., 1984).

The same group of authors reported that the chemical was clearly absorbed through the skin. The time span until the onset of death ($TL_{50}$), which was measured in the muscles, was 2 hours (no further details; Chalepo et al., 1984).

## 8. Experience in humans

No information available.

## 9. Threshold limit values

The TLV value in the USSR is 0.01 mg/m$^3$ air, with the risk phrases "penetrates the skin, dangerous substance class I" (Chalepo et al., 1984).

## References

Bayer AG, Institut für Toxikologie
p-Chlorbenzotrichlorid – Gewerbetoxikologische Untersuchungen
Unpublished report No. 9063 (1980a)

Bayer AG, Institut für Toxikologie
p-Chlorbenzotrichlorid – Untersuchung zur akuten oralen Toxizität an männlichen Wistar-Ratten
Unpublished report of 1. 8. 1980b

Chalepo, A.I., Veselovskaja, K.A., Lapina, L.M., Popova, S.M., Voroncov, R.S.
Materialien zur Begründung der maximal zulässigen Konzentration von $\alpha,\alpha,\alpha$-Trichlor-4-chlortoluol in der Luft am Arbeitsplatz
Gig. Tr. Prof. Zabol., 6, 41–43 (1984)

Fukuda, K., Matsushita, H., Takemoto, K.
Kanzerogenese von p-Chlorbenzotrichlorid
52nd Ann. Meeting, Japan Assoc. Ind. Health, p. 330 (1979) and English translation of the original report
Communicated by Hoechst Japan (1988)

Hoechst AG, Pharma Forschung Toxikologie
p-Chlorbenzotrichlorid – Prüfung der akuten oralen Toxizität an der männlichen und weiblichen Wistar-Ratte
Unpublished report No. 84.0041 (1984)

Hoechst AG, Pharma Research Toxicology
Study of the mutagenic potential in strains of *Salmonella typhimurium* (Ames Test) and *Escherichia coli*
Report No. 86.1462 (1986)

Hoechst AG, Pharma Forschung Toxikologie
p-Chlorbenzotrichlorid TTR – Prüfung der akuten dermalen Toxizität an der Wistar-Ratte
Unpublished report No. 88.0121 (1988a)

Hoechst AG, Pharma Research Toxicology and Pathology
p-Chlorbenzotrichlorid TTR, Detection of gene mutations in somatic cells in culture, HGPRT-test with V79 cells
Unpublished report No. 88.0932 (1988b)

Hoechst AG
Data sheet "Altstoffe", May 1989

Matsushita, H., Fukuda, K., Takemoto, K.
Carcinogenicity of benzotrichloride and its related compounds
Hoechst AG, unpublished report No. 76/0729 (1977)

Quistad, G.B., Mulholland, K.M., Skiles, G., Jamieson, G.C.
Metabolism of 4-chlorobenzotrichloride in rats
J. Agric. Food Chem., 33 (1) 95–98 (1985)

Schreiber, G.
Bericht über die Prüfung von p-Chlorbenzotrichlorid 99 auf primäre Hautreizwirkung
Fraunhofer-Institut für Toxikologie and Aerosolforschung (1980a)
Commissioned by Bayer AG

Schreiber, G.
Bericht über die Prüfung von p-Chlorbenzotrichlorid 99 auf Schleimhautreizwirkung
Fraunhofer-Institut für Toxikologie und Aerosolforschung (1980b)
Commissioned by Bayer AG

# Compound chemical index vol. 1–3

Acetylene carbinol *2*, 121
Acrylic acid *2*, 41
Adipic acid dinitrile *1*, 252
Adiponitrile *1*, 252
Adipyl dinitrile *1*, 252
AH *1*, 182
2-Amino-1-methoxy-4-nitrobenzene *1*, 155
1-Amino-2-methyl-4-nitrobenzene *2*, 101
1-Amino-3-nitrobenzene *2*, 88
1-Amino-4-chloro-2-nitrobenzene *1*, 75
1-Amino-4-methoxy-2-methylbenzene *1*, 173
2-Amino-5-chloro-nitrobenzene *1*, 75
2-Amino-5-nitrotoluene *2*, 101
2,2′-Aminodiethanol *2*, 136
m-Aminonitrobenzene *2*, 88
3-Aminonitrobenzene *2*, 88
Ammonyx 200 *1*, 312
Ansibases Red RL *2*, 101
Arasan *3*, 93
asym-dimethyl ethylene *2*, 153
Azoamine Scarlet K *1*, 155
Azoene Fast Red GL Base *2*, 101
Azogene Fast Red RL *2*, 101
Azoic Diazo Component 13, Base *1*, 155

Benzene-1,4-dicarbonic acid *3*, 48
1,4-Benzene dicarbonic acid *3*, 47
1,4-Benzene dicarbonic acid dimethyl ester *1*, 266
1,4-Benzene dicarboxylic acid *3*, 48
p-Benzene dicarboxylic acid *3*, 48
1,4-Benzene dicarboxylic acid dimethyl ester *1*, 267
1,2-benzodicarbonitrile *2*, 76
p-Benzoquinone monooxime *2*, 108
1,4-Benzoquinone oxime *2*, 108
N,N′-Bis(1-methylpropyl)-1,4-benzenediamine *1*, 166
N,N′-Bis(1-methylpropyl)-1,4-diaminobenzene *1*, 166
Bis-(dimethylthiocarbamoyl) disulphide *3*, 93
Bis(2,3-epoxypropyl)-ether *3*, 156
BLO *1*, 134
Braunstein *1*, 329
Brecolane NDG *1*, 219
Bromoform *3*, 2
Butane dinitrile *1*, 252
1,4-Butanolide *1*, 134
But(2)ene-1,4-dicarboxylic acid dimethyl ester *2*, 169
Butyl ethyl acetaldehyde *2*, 161
Butyl phosphate *1*, 298
α-butylene *2*, 153
γ-butylene *2*, 153
i-butylene *2*, 153
2-Butyne-1,4-diol *1*, 207
Butynediol *1*, 207

Butyric acid 4-hydroxy-,
gamma-lactone *1*, 134
Butyric acid lactone *1*, 134
4-Butyrolactone *1*, 134
Butyryl lactone *1*, 134

CAEE *1*, 319
CAS-No.
75-02-5 *2*, 1
75-25-2 *3*, 2
78-83-1 *1*, 44
78-79-5 *2*, 14
79-07-2 *1*, 59
79-10-7 *2*, 41
88-10-8 *3*, 19
88-16-4 *3*, 27
89-63-4 *1*, 75
91-15-6 *2*, 76
96-34-4 *3*, 33
96-45-7 *1*, 83
96-48-0 *1*, 134
98-15-7 *3*, 41
99-59-2 *1*, 155
99-09-2 *2*, 88
99-52-5 *2*, 101
100-21-0 *3*, 47
101-96-2 *1*, 166
102-50-1 *1*, 173
104-76-7 *1*, 182
104-91-6 *2*, 108
107-19-7 *2*, 121
109-59-1 *3*, 61
110-65-6 *1*, 207
111-42-2 *2*, 136
111-46-6 *1*, 219
111-69-3 *1*, 252
115-11-7 *2*, 153
120-61-6 *1*, 266
122-60-1 *3*, 74
123-51-3 *1*, 284
123-05-7 *2*, 161
126-73-8 *1*, 298
137-26-8 *3*, 93
138-24-9 *1*, 311
541-41-3 *1*, 319
624-48-6 *2*, 169
625-45-6 *3*, 132
935-92-2 *2*, 178
1313-13-9 *1*, 328
2044-88-4 *2*, 185
2136-89-2 *3*, 147
2238-07-5 *3*, 156
2243-62-1 *2*, 192
5216-25-1 *3*, 168
Celluphos 4 *1*, 298
Chloressigsäuremethylester
*3*, 34
2-Chloro-1-trichloro-methylbenzene *3*, 147
4-Chloro-1-trichloro-methylbenzene *3*, 168
4-Chloro-2-nitroaniline *1*, 75
Chloroacetamide *1*, 59
α-Chloroacetamide *1*, 60
2-Chloroacetamide *1*, 59
Chloroacetic acid amide
*1*, 60
Chloroacetic acid methyl
ester *3*, 33
p-Chlorbenzotrichlorid *3*, 168
o-Chlorobenzotrichloride *3*,
147
p-Chlorobenzotrichloride *3*,
168
4-Chlorobenzotrichloride *3*,
168
m-Chlorobenzotrifluoride *3*,
41
o-Chlorobenzotrifluoride *1*, 27
2-Chlorobenzotrifluoride *3*, 27
3-Chlorobenzotrifluoride *3*, 41

Chloroformic acid ethyl ester *1*, 319
p-Chloro-o-nitroaniline *1*, 75
3-Chlor-α,α,α-trifluortoluol *3*, 41
2-Chloro-α,α,α-trifluorotoluene *3*, 27
3-Chloro-α,α,α-trifluorotoluene *3*, 41
2-Chloro-1-trifluoro-methylbenzene *3*, 27
3-Chloro-1-trifluoromethylbenzene *3*, 41
C.I. 37030 *2*, 88
CNA *1*, 75
m-Cresidine *1*, 173

Daito Red Base RL *2*, 101
DEA *2*, 136
Deactivator E *1*, 219
Deactivator H *1*, 219
DEG *1*, 219
DGE *3*, 156
Devol Red RL *2*, 101
Diabase Red RL *2*, 101
1,5-Diaminonaphthalene *2*, 192, 193
DICOL *1*, 219
o-dicyanobenzene *2*, 76
1,2-dicyanobenzol *2*, 76
1,4-Dicyanobutane *1*, 252
Di(2,3-epoxypropyl)ether *3*, 156
Diethanolamine *2*, 136
N,N-Diethanolamine *2*, 136
Diethylcarbamic acid chloride *3*, 19
Diethylcarbamidsäurechlorid *3*, 19
Diethylcarbamoylchlorid *3*, 19
Diethylcarbamoyl chloride *3*, 19
N,N-Diethylcarbamoyl chloride *3*, 19
Diethylene glycol *1*, 219
Diethylolamine *2*, 136
Diglycidyl ether *3*, 156
Diglycol *1*, 219
Dihydro-2(3H)-furanone *1*, 133
4,5-Dihydro-2-mercaptoimidazole *1*, 83
beta,beta′-Dihydroxydiethyl ether *1*, 219
2,2′-Dihydroxy-diethylamine *2*, 136
β,β′-Dihydroxy-diethylamine *2*, 136
Dimethyl-1,4-benzene dicarboxylate *1*, 267
Dimethyl maleate *2*, 169
Dimethyl terephthalate *1*, 266
Dimethylmaleinat *2*, 169
Dimethyl-p-phthalate *1*, 267
2,4-Dinitro-1-methyl-aminobenzene *2*, 185
2,4-Dinitromethylaniline *2*, 185
2,4-Dinitro-N-methylaniline *2*, 185
But-2-yne-1,4-diol *1*, 207
Diolamine *2*, 136
1,4-Dioxy-butyne-2 *1*, 207
N,N′-Di-sec.-butyl-p-phenylenediamine *1*, 166
Disflamol 1 TB *1*, 298
Dissolvand APU *1*, 219
DMM *2*, 169
DMT *1*, 267
DuPont Gasoline Antioxidant No. 22 *1*, 166

1,2-Epoxy-3-phenoxy-
propane *3*, 74
2,3-Epoxypropylphenyl ether
*3*, 74
Ethanol, 2,2′-oxydi- *1*, 219
Ethene carboxylic acid *2*, 41
Z-Ethene dicarboxylic
acid dimethyl ester *2*, 169
Ethenyl methanol *2*, 121
Ethylbutylacetaldehyde
*2*, 162
2-Ethylcaproaldehyde *2*, 161
α-Ethylcaproaldehyde *2*, 162
Ethylchlorocarbonate *1*, 319
Ethylchloroformiate *1*, 319
Ethylchloromethanate *1*, 319
Ethylene carboxylic acid *2*, 42
Ethylene diglycol *1*, 219
Ethylene glycol isopropyl
ether *3*, 62
Ethylene glycol monoisopropyl
ether *3*, 62
Ethylene thiourea *1*, 83
Ethylenethiourea *1*, 83
N,N′-Ethylenethiourea *1*, 83
1,3-Ethylenethiourea *1*, 83
Ethylhexaldehyde *2*, 162
2-Ethylhexaldehyde *2*, 162
2-Ethylhexan-1-ol *1*, 182
2-Ethylhexanal *2*, 161
2-Ethylhexanol-1 *1*, 182
2-Ethylhexanol *1*, 182
2-Ethylhexyl alcohol *1*, 182
Ethynyl carbinol *2*, 121
ETU *1*, 83

Fast Red 5NT *2*, 101
Fast Red RL Base *2*, 101
Fernacol *3*, 93
Fernasan *3*, 93
Fluoroethylene *2*, 1

gamma-BL *1*, 134
gamma-Butyrolactone *1*, 133
GBL *1*, 134
Glycidyl phenyl ether *3*, 74
Glycol ether *1*, 219
Glycol ethyl ether *1*, 219
Golpanol *1*, 207

Hemiterpene *2*, 14
Hexanedioic acid dinitrile
*1*, 252
Hiltonil Fast Red RL Base
*2*, 102
1-Hydroxy-4-nitrosobenzene
*2*, 108
4-Hydroxybutanoic acid lac-
tone *1*, 134
4-Hydroxybutanoic acid,
gamma-lactone *1*, 134
gamma-Hydroxybutyric acid
cyclic ester *1*, 134
gamma-Hydroxybutyric acid
lactone *1*, 134
4-Hydroxybutyric acid lac-
tone *1*, 134
4-Hydroxybutyric acid, gamma-
lactone *1*, 134
Bis-(2-hydroxyethyl)amine
*2*, 136
Di-(2-hydroxyethyl)amine
*2*, 136
Bis(2-hydroxyethyl)ether
*1*, 219
β-Hydroxyethyl isopropyl
ether *3*, 62
1-Hydroxymethylpropane
*1*, 44

Imidazolidinethione *1*, 83
2-Imidazolidinethione *1*, 83
Imidazoline-2(3H)-thione *1*, 83

Imidazoline-2-thiol *1*, 83
2,2′-Iminobisethanol *2*, 136
IPEGE *3*, 62
Isoamyl alcohol *1*, 284
Isobutanol *1*, 44
isobutene *2*, 153
Isobutyl alcohol *1*, 44
Isobutylcarbinol *1*, 284
isobutylene *2*, 153
Isoctanol *1*, 182
Isopentyl alcohol *1*, 284
Isoprene *2*, 14
2-Isopropoxyethanol *3*, 62
Isopropyl Cellosolve *3*, 62
Isopropyl ethylene glycol ether *3*, 61
Isopropylethylenglykolether *3*, 62
Isopropyl glycol *3*, 62

Kako Red RL Base *2*, 102
Kayaku Red RL Base *2*, 102
Kerobit BPD *1*, 166
Korantin BH *1*, 207, 209

MAA *3*, 132
MAD *2*, 169
Maleic acid dimethyl ester *2*, 169
Manganese dioxide *1*, 328
Meisei Fast Red RL Base *2*, 102
2-Mercapto-2-imidazoline *1*, 83
Mercaptoimidazoline *1*, 83
Mercazin 1 NA 22 *1*, 83
Methenyltribromide *3*, 2
Methoxyacetic acid *3*, 132
2-Methoxyacetic acid *3*, 132
Methoxyessigsäure *3*, 132
4-Methoxy-2-methylaniline *1*, 173
4-Methoxy-2-methylbenzen amine *1*, 174
2-Methoxy-5-nitroaniline *1*, 155
2-Methoxy-5-nitrobenzen amine *1*, 155
Methyl-4-carbomethoxy-benzoate *1*, 267
2-(1-Methylethoxy)-ethanol *3*, 62
2-Methyl-4-methoxyaniline *1*, 174
2-Methyl-4-nitroaniline *2*, 101
2-Methyl-4-nitrobenzenamine *2*, 101
2-Methyl-1,3-butadiene *2*, 14
N-Methyl-2,4-dinitroaniline *2*, 185
N-Methyl-2,4-dinitrobenzen-amine *2*, 185
β-Methyl bivinyl *2*, 14
Methyl maleate *2*, 169
Bis-oxy methylacetylene *1*, 207
Methylbutadiene-1,3 *2*, 14
3-Methylbutanol-1 *1*, 284
Methylchloroacetate *3*, 34
Methylmonochloroacetate *3*, 34
2-Methyl-p-anisidine *1*, 173
4-Methyl-3-oxapentan-1-ol *3*, 61
2-Methylpropan-1-ol *1*, 44
2-Methylpropane-1-ol *1*, 44
2-Methylpropanol-1 *1*, 44
2-Methylpropene *2*, 153
2-Methylpropyl alcohol *1*, 44
Microcide Mergal AF *1*, 60
2,2′-Iminodiethanol *2*, 136
Mitsui Red RL Base *2*, 102
Monofluoroethylene *2*, 1

1,5-Naphthalene diamine *2*, 193
1,5-Naphthyl diamine *2*, 193
1,5-Naphthylendiamin *2*, 193
1,5-Naphthylene diamine *2*, 192
Naphtoelan Red RL Base *2*, 102
NCI-C55878 *1*, 134
m-Nitranilin *2*, 88
5-Nitro-2-aminotoluene *2*, 101
m-Nitroaminobenzene *2*, 88
3-Nitroaniline *2*, 88
m-Nitroaniline *2*, 88
5-Nitroanisidine *1*, 155
3-Nitrobenzenamine *2*, 88
5-Nitro-ortho-anisidine *1*, 155
4-Nitro-o-toluidine *2*, 101
p-Nitro-o-toluidine *2*, 101
m-Nitrophenylamine *2*, 88
p-Nitrosophenol *2*, 108
4-Nitrosophenol *2*, 108

Octanol, technical *1*, 182
Octyl aldehyde *2*, 162
3-Oxa-1,5-pentanediol *1*, 219
3-Oxapentane-1,5-diol *1*, 219
Oxitol *3*, 62
2,2′-Oxybisethanol *1*, 220
2,2′-Oxydiethanol TL4N *1*, 220
o-PDN *2*, 76

Pennac CRA *1*, 83
PGE *3*, 74
Phenylglycidyl ether *3*, 74
Phenyltrimethyl-ammonium chloride *1*, 311
Phenoxymethyloxirane *3*, 74
Phenoxypropene oxide *3*, 74
Phosphoric acid tri-n-butyl-ester *1*, 298
phthalic acid dinitrile *2*, 76
o-phthalodinitrile (o-PDN) *2*, 76
phthalodinitrile *2*, 76
Pomasol *3*, 93
Pomarsol *3*, 93
Propargyl alcohol *2*, 121
2-Propenoic acid *2*, 42
Propyne-(1)-ol-(3) *2*, 121
2-Propyne-1-ol *2*, 121
Propyne-(2)-ol *2*, 121
1-Propyne-3-ol *2*, 121
2-Propynol-1 *2*, 121
p-Pseudocumoquinone *2*, 178
Pyrolusite *1*, 329

p-Quinone monooxime *2*, 108
Quinone oxime *2*, 108

Red Base Ciba X *2*, 102
Red Base Irga X *2*, 102
Red Base NRL *2*, 102
Red RL Base *2*, 102
Rhenogram ETU *1*, 83
Rhodanin S 62 *1*, 83

Sipomer *2*, 169
Soxinol 22 *1*, 83
Spectrolene Red RL *2*, 102
Symulon Red RL Base *2*, 102

TBP *1*, 298
Tenamene 2 *1*, 166
Terephthalic acid *3*, 47
Terephthalic acid dimethyl ester *1*, 267

Terephthalsäure *3*, 48
Tersan *3*, 93
α,α,α,2-Tetrachlorotoluene *3*, 147
α,α,α,4-Tetrachlorotoluene *3*, 168
α,α,α,2-Tetrachlortoluol *3*,147
Tetramethylene cyanide *1*, 252
Tetramethylene dicyanide *1*, 252
Tetramethylthiuram disulphide *3*, 93
Thiosan *3*, 93
Thiotex *3*, 93
Thiourea, N,N′-(1,2-ethandiyl) *1*, 83
Thiram *3*, 93
Thiuram *3*, 93
TMTD *3*, 93
TPA *3*, 48
TPS *3*, 48
Tribromomethane *3*, 2
Tributyl phosphate *1*, 298
α,α,α-Trichloro-2-chlorotoluene *3*, 147
α,α,α-Trichloro-4-chlorotoluene *3*, 168
Tri-n-butyl phosphate *1*, 298
2,3,5-Trimethyl-2,5-cyclohexadiene-1,4-dione *2*, 178
Trimethylanilinium chloride *1*, 312
N,N,N-Trimethylbenzen-ammonium chloride *1*, 311
Trimethylbenzoquinone *2*, 178
Trimethylchinon *2*, 178
2,3,5-Trimethylcyclohexa-2,5-diene-1,4-dione *2*, 178
2,3,5-Trimethyl-p-benzoquinone *2*, 178
Trimethylphenyl ammonium chloride *1*, 311
Trimethylquinone *2*, 178
2,3,6-Trimethylquinone *2*, 178
Tulabase Fast Red RL *2*, 102

VF *2*, 1
Vinyl carboxylic acid *2*, 42
Vinyl fluoride *2*, 1, 2
Vulcacit NPV/C *1*, 83
Vulkacit Thiuram *3*, 93

Warecure C *1*, 83

Yamada Fast Red RL Base *2*, 102